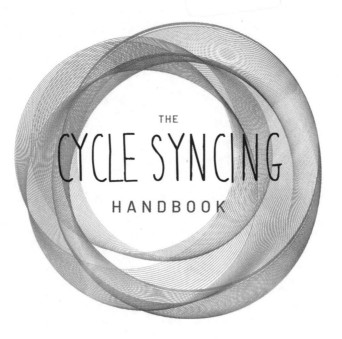

THE

CYCLE SYNCING

HANDBOOK

IDENTIFY HORMONAL PATTERNS, BUILD HOLISTIC HABITS,
AND EMBRACE THE POWER OF YOUR MENSTRUAL CYCLE

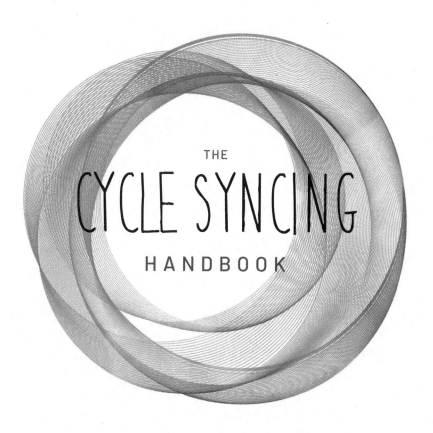

THE

CYCLE SYNCING

HANDBOOK

ANGIE MARIE

Published by:
Ulysses Press
PO Box 3440
Berkeley, CA 94703
www.ulyssespress.com

ISBN: 978-1-64604-560-0
Library of Congress Control Number: 2023938338

Printed in the United States by Kingery Printing Company
10 9 8 7 6 5 4 3 2 1

Acquisitions editor: Claire Sielaff
Project editor: Renee Rutledge
Managing editor: Claire Chun
Proofreader: Barbara Schultz
Front cover design: Rebecca Lown
Interior design and layout: Winnie Liu

IMPORTANT NOTE TO READERS: This book has been written and published for informational and educational purposes only. It is not intended to serve as medical advice or to be any form of medical treatment. You should always consult with your physician before altering or changing any aspect of your medical treatment. Do not stop or change any prescription medications without the guidance and advice of your physician. Any use of the information in this book is made on the reader's good judgment and is the reader's sole responsibility. This book is not intended to diagnose or treat any medical condition and is not a substitute for a physician. This book is independently authored and published and no sponsorship or endorsement of this book by, and no affiliation with, any trademarked brands or other products mentioned within is claimed or suggested. All trademarks that appear in this book belong to their respective owners and are used here for informational purposes only. The author and publisher encourage readers to patronize the brands mentioned in this book.

CONTENTS

● ● ●

WE ARE NOT ROBOTS

● ● ●

If you opened this book, then you have an inkling of an idea that your menstrual cycle is important enough to learn about. What you—and the world—need to know is that the menstrual cycle's effects go far beyond reproduction. In fact, in 2016, the American College of Obstetricians and Gynecologists named the menstrual cycle to be a vital sign, just like pulse and body temperature.[1]

Yet, modern society teaches us to neglect, suppress, and hide our menstrual cycles, even though the cycle is intertwined with the function of the whole body. Your brain, metabolism, microbiome, stress response, immune system and, of course, reproductive cycle are all closely linked to your fertility.

Society conditioned us menstruators to cringe at period talk, stuff our tampons to the bottom of our bags in fear others will see them, and blame any negative mood on "PMS." The reality? Your period—or rather, your entire menstrual cycle—holds vital clues to your health and immense wisdom around your wellness.

YOUR INNER RHYTHMS MATTER

The human body relies on many cycles to function and thrive. However, not all cycles work on the same time frame. **Circadian rhythms** are processes that occur on a 24-hour basis, like the sleep-wake cycle. **Ultradian rhythms** occur repeatedly within 24 hours, such as sleep stages, appetite, and blood circulation. And **infradian rhythms** last longer than 24 hours. These cycles work in

. . . .
1 Committee on Adolescent Health Care, "Menstruation in Girls and Adolescents: Using the Menstrual Cycle as a Vital Sign," American College of Obstetricians and Gynecologists, December 2015, https://www.acog.org/clinical/clinical-guidance/committee-opinion/articles/2015/12/menstruation-in-girls-and-adolescents-using-the-menstrual-cycle-as-a-vital-sign.

synergy to ensure you survive and, hopefully, thrive. By ignoring the infradian rhythm of the menstrual cycle, we put body systems at risk of not working optimally, and the effects don't feel good.

Think about how you feel when your circadian rhythm gets screwed up, like if you get jet lag, or have a rough night's sleep, or spend a week in Alaska during summer when it's sunny at night. You typically feel groggy and tired and may even experience stomach or mood problems. In a similar way, when other cycles fall out of whack, including your menstrual cycle, you can end up feeling unwell. Think about a stressful month at work, when your premenstrual symptoms are way worse than usual, or if your menstrual cycle disappears completely due to poor nutrition and you have no energy to do the sports you love anymore.

Your body's many cycles dictate how you feel, and cycles are inherently made up of a process of *change*. The levels of hormones that run the menstrual cycle *change* over the course of a cycle. Because of this built-in cyclical nature, we as humans with menstrual cycles can't realistically expect to show up the same exact way day after day. That would be fighting our very biology! We are cyclical beings, and there's no changing that. We are not robots.

LINEAR VS CYCLICAL LIVING

Unfortunately, the structure of society is built primarily on a 24-hour cycle. Office workers typically stay at work from 8 a.m. to 5 p.m. every day, no matter their energy levels. Our social media feeds are full of highlights, as if everybody is always at peak happiness. Workout and nutrition plans often recommend a "same thing every day" approach. The idea of productivity is so often reliant on what you do in a *day*, when in reality, most parts of life, like exercise, seasonal nutrition, the creative process, and so on (all of which we'll discuss in this book) more naturally flow in phases.

When people repeat the same habits in the same way day after day, it could be called **linear living**. They might eat the same breakfast every day, clock into work at the same time every day to plow through the same tasks, force themselves through the same workout that doesn't actually sound appealing that day, etc. This isn't to say that habits and structure are *bad*, but all too often, our linear-leaning standards set us up to ignore our bodies' nudges when it comes to managing health and happiness. Your body and mind might be screaming for something different—whether it's the nutrients in your food, the benefits of a

THE CYCLE SYNCING HANDBOOK

different workout, or a new creative endeavor—but we're conditioned to tamp down any feelings of discontent for the sake of the hustle and grind.

There's another way, which I call **cyclical living**. It might not look drastically different from linear living from the outside, but it can make all the difference in how you approach your habits, work, self-care, and beyond. Cyclical living involves adapting your schedule, actions, and routines in order to best fit what your body needs at that particular time.

You might cycle through four different morning routines over the course of the month, switching every week. You might change your workouts periodically to incorporate times of building and times of rest (rather than pushing yourself at the same moderate intensity day after day). You can plan ahead for how you anticipate you'll energetically feel on a certain weekend, so you can avoid committing to plans you won't feel up to when the day arrives, and instead schedule social activities for when you know you'll feel most up for it.

Linear living says, "If you try hard enough, you might be able to have it all someday!" Cyclical living says, "You can have it all—just not all at once."

Linear living says, "Get better at time management and you'll get more done." Cyclical living says, "Manage your energy, not your time."

Linear living says, "You're stuck because you're unmotivated and need to push yourself through the resistance." Cyclical living says, "You know that you'll be better suited for that task next week, and right now is better for the other task."

Realistically, given the way our world is structured, we'll always have *some* amount of linear living built into our lives. But what if we could work just a bit more in harmony with our bodies by tapping into cyclical living practices where we can?

CYCLE SYNCING: CYCLICAL LIVING THROUGH THE MENSTRUAL CYCLE

Turns out, cyclical living can come pretty naturally to many of us. The menstrual cycle acts as a built-in blueprint for living cyclically over the days, weeks, and months. With half the people on Earth experiencing periods at some point in life, and with every human's reason for existing being owed to the menstrual cycle, our physiology itself holds immense wisdom for living with more harmony across our busy lives.

The concept of **cycle syncing** describes a framework and set of tools for people with periods, who I call "menstruators," to align their nutrition, fitness, work, creativity, relationships, and hobbies to their menstrual cycle. The menstrual cycle is composed of four phases due to changing hormone levels, and each phase lends itself to a way of living that can optimize how you think, feel, and perform.

When you can work *with* your physiology to identify your needs and desires for any given day and week—rather than expecting them to be unchanging—you can move, eat, work, and play in a way that feels happier, healthier, and easier.

Have you ever noticed that some weeks you're on fire, banging out the whole to-do list, but then the next week, you can't focus at all on those same tasks? Or that some weeks you kick butt exercising at high intensity and feel super strong, but then the next week you feel like you can't keep up? Maybe you snap at your partner a few days a month and just blame it on PMS, or you crave avocados for a week but then can't bring yourself to finish the rest before they rot?

These are all clues from your body's hormonal changes, manifesting as a change in what you desire and how you feel. If you learn how to decode the clues, you can be proactive and reactive to your current cycle phase and primed to feel optimally well. Cycle syncing helps you honor those cyclical patterns, give yourself grace for not showing up the exact same way day after day, and notice what you feel, want, and need in each unique day.

And if you're not currently having periods? That's okay you can still use a cycle syncing framework! Whether you're on hormonal birth control, are postpartum, or no longer get periods, you can learn to live cyclically without true menstrual cycles. (I cover this subject in more detail toward the end of this book.)

You'll likely feel healthiest and happiest living a lifestyle that accounts for your menstrual cycle, and once you understand how and why your cycles work, you'll feel more motivated to implement positive change and make progress toward your goals. This book intends to help you enhance your own life by tapping into that beautiful internal rhythm that we all too often dismiss as "just a period." Turns out, there's a lot more behind it than a few days of bleeding each month!

Cyclical living doesn't have to be complicated. Actually, it'll eventually come easy. Nature designed you to be a strong and efficient leader, connector, and creator, and in this book we'll dig into how to use those powers.

THE PILLARS OF CYCLE SYNCING

As you start on this journey, keep in mind these guiding pillars of cycle syncing. They'll remind you of what's most important when you run into obstacles or opportunities.

MANAGE YOUR ENERGY, NOT YOUR TIME

We're inundated with articles on how to boost our productivity, apps that promise to magically get us back more time in the day, and celebrities who endorse start-and-stop habits that we hope will somehow cure our woes when it comes to not having enough time in the day. I'm not saying that some of those resources aren't valuable, but I do think we need to shift some of the focus to managing our energy instead of our time.

We can have it all. We just can't have it all *at once*. By tuning in to our shifting energy levels, we can notice when we are best primed to do certain tasks and creatively schedule them in a way that will actually increase efficiency and help us get more done with less resistance.

As you start cycle syncing, I hope that you'll consider the questions "What is the most effective thing I could do today based on my energy?" and "How could I arrange my to-dos in a way that feels good to my mind and body right now?" rather than "Why can't I find a daily routine that I can stick to every single day?" or " What's the silver bullet for finishing my entire to-do list in one day?"

PLAY OVER PERFECTION

Living cyclically is about experimenting. There's no way to "win" cycle syncing. The point of living cyclically is to feel better in the day to day. If you impose a bunch of strict rules on yourself, you're setting yourself up to feel bad when you can't follow them perfectly.

Instead, cycle syncing is supposed to be fun! It's supposed to give you reasons to try new things, follow your curiosities, bring projects to completion, and learn what to scrap. Cycle syncing helps you release guilt because it reminds you that there is no one fail-proof method to live in harmony with all of your responsibilities. Rather, it's about playing with different ideas and seeing what works for you, right now.

Change is the only constant. So why not have fun and experiment with that, instead of trying to force your life to be the same every day? You have permission to change your habits, ideas, and lifestyle over time, so play with it and release the urge of perfectionism.

YOUR EXPERIENCE ABOVE ALL

No framework is universal. Your lived experience outshines any idea or template created or followed by somebody else.

More than anything, cycle syncing is a framework for you to acknowledge and honor your lived experiences beyond any suggested patterns I outline in this book. If your cyclical experience differs from others, that is great! What matters is that you feel literate in reading your body and its cues.

Release the pressure to force your body to feel something it doesn't or act in a way it doesn't want to. Your inner seasons might manifest differently from mine, and mine might manifest differently from those of your friends. You might even find you enjoy some aspects of linear living more than cyclical living, and that's okay. Your lived experience matters more than the words in a book.

Although everybody's cycle and cyclical experience is unique, everyone I've spoken with about it has agreed that it positively affects their life in some way. A few examples:

❀ "Maybe it's a bit cliché, but cycle syncing taught me to not get attached to my highest highs or my lowest lows. Because in reality, everything is temporary and going to change soon." —Shelley

❀ "It was only through tracking my cycle that I recognized the connection between the phase of my cycle and symptom flares of my chronic illness. I'm still working out the finer points, but even just understanding that my cycle impacts how I feel health-wise has led to a lot less frustration." —Rachel

❀ "As I started to understand the hormonal and physical changes I go through, I began to let go of this idea that there must be something wrong with me. Changes came to be expected and something to work with instead of fight against. Not only did it improve the relationship I had with myself and my body, but also with my intimate relationship with my partner." —Kelly

DISCLAIMERS BEFORE YOU START

As you begin your journey of cycle syncing, I urge you to seek medical advice from the appropriate individuals when needed. I am not a medical care provider and do not offer medical advice. If you have concerns around your body or cycle, seek care from a qualified medical professional. However, a perk of tracking your cycle—especially signs of ovulation and the characteristics of your period—is that it can provide data that can help your doctor arrive at a diagnosis or test recommendations.

Also, I'd like to acknowledge the privilege I hold as a white, cisgender woman whose intersections of race, gender, class, and ability are often to my benefit. I share the tools in this book with you from my own life experiences and those of my clients; this may leave out certain perspectives of which I'm not yet aware. Please be mindful to take what resonates with you, and leave the rest.

The more you can interpret your own unique patterns, the fewer negative effects you'll feel from outside influences. The more you can listen to your inner wisdom and know who and how you are, the more confident you'll feel in taking action in all areas of your life. The more you can embrace the beauty of living as a cyclical being, the more society's stigma will lessen around periods. And that's how future generations will begin to see their cycles as a symbol of power, not oppression.

WAIT A SEC! PREREQUISITES TO CYCLE SYNCING

Before we dig into how to start cycle syncing, I'll walk you through the basic anatomy and physiology of the menstrual cycle. (Don't worry, it'll be painless compared to middle school.)

Then, I'll introduce the four phases of the menstrual cycle and how they align with four inner seasons as the framework for living cyclically.

The meat of the book will be how you can move, eat, work, play, and create while playing to the strengths of your inner seasons and managing the challenges that may arise in each.

Finally, I'll address common obstacles that could pop up and how to make cycle syncing work with your life so you can continue on your powerful way.

So buckle up. Let's get cyclical.

CHAPTER 1

GET TO KNOW YOUR FLOW

• • •

Think back to your middle school health class. (Cringe, I know.) Was it a disaster, like in the movie *Mean Girls* when the teacher says "Don't have sex, because you will get pregnant and die"? Did the teacher pass around a condom, but never a menstrual cup? Or maybe it was just... awkward. It probably heavily focused on menstrual *periods* as opposed to an entire cycle, and specifically addressed how to handle bleeding.

In fact, most people could tell you far more about tampon and pad options than about the actual biological forces at play. But in order to understand cycle syncing, you first need to know the basics of anatomy and physiology when it comes to your reproductive system.

Let's take a simple (but *finally* accurate) peek into our bodies' internal plumbing.

MENSTRUAL CYCLE ANATOMY

UTERUS: THE MAIN VESSEL, THE WOMB

Your uterus is a hollow organ in your lower abdomen, located between your bladder and rectum. It's pear-shaped and about the size of a small lemon when you're not pregnant—but becomes watermelon-sized in late pregnancy!

The uterus builds up a blood-rich lining and releases it by having a period at the end of every cycle in which pregnancy doesn't occur. And if conception does occur? The uterus becomes the home of the fetus.

ENDOMETRIUM: THE INNER LINING OF THE UTERUS

This lining of the uterus is called the endometrium. It builds up to prepare a nice and cozy spot for a fertilized egg and eventual fetus, then sheds itself as your period if you don't become pregnant that cycle. In other words, period blood is a mixture of endometrial blood and tissue (plus water and mucus).

CERVIX: THE BOTTOM OF THE UTERUS

The cervix is at the bottom of the uterus, low enough that you can feel it yourself! It contains channels, called crypts, that produce fluid to help sperm live. You see this fluid throughout your cycle; it's most obvious during the fertile days of the cycle.

The cervical os is the small opening in the cervix that gets bigger around ovulation to allow sperm in, and it *really* expands during childbirth—to about 10 centimeters!

VAGINA: THE CANAL BETWEEN THE CERVIX AND VULVA

The vagina is a muscular passage, about four to six inches long. It's elastic, so it can expand during intercourse and childbirth. Pro tip: The vagina is internal, the vulva is external. Many people mistakenly say "vagina" to describe the external anatomy, including the labia and clitoris, when they actually mean vulva.

OVARIES: THE EGG-MAKERS NEXT TO THE UTERUS

The two almond-sized ovaries are sex glands that house a ton of immature eggs. You were born with all the eggs you'd ever have, around one to two million! The ovaries contain small, fluid-filled sacs called follicles that produce hormones that drive the cycle.

Ova are eggs stored in your ovaries. Between puberty and menopause, one egg, called an ovum, is released per cycle (out of 15 to 20 contenders), and this release is called **ovulation**. In rare cases where more than one egg is released, you end up with fraternal twins (or more).

You're only fertile the handful of days around ovulation, meaning... drumroll please... you can't get pregnant every day of the cycle!

The coolest egg fact? If you become pregnant, your developing fetus is already carrying their eggs—which means you're carrying eggs that could become your grandchildren, too!

FALLOPIAN TUBES: THE PASSAGEWAYS BETWEEN THE UTERUS AND OVARIES

When you ovulate, the egg is drawn toward one of the two narrow fallopian tubes, which are about four to five inches long. If conception does not occur, the egg disintegrates. If a sperm travels up to fertilize an egg in the tube, then the fertilized egg continues down to get to its new home in the uterus.

THE BRAIN: THE HORMONE-SIGNALLING CENTER

We won't dive into all the processes, but I'd be remiss to ignore the brain's role altogether. Your hypothalamus and pituitary gland send signals that lead to the production of hormones that we'll get to in a moment.

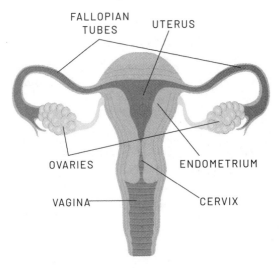

THE GIST OF IT

Let's make it super-duper simple: Your egg follicles grow as your cervix creates fluid and opens up, making you fertile. The ovary releases an egg, which travels down a tube and tumbles into the uterus. When your hormones signal that you're not pregnant, the endometrium sheds, and blood exits through the vagina.

See? Easy peasy. It's key to understand your anatomy so that you can then learn the physiology—where the real magic happens.

MENSTRUAL CYCLE PHYSIOLOGY

Speaking of hormones... what exactly are they? **Hormones** are your body's chemical messengers. Glands in your body release hormones into your bloodstream so they can send a message to another part of the body, telling it what to do or how you should behave. They control every process your body does, from digestion and sleep to heart rate and mood. So when someone says, "Ugh, you're acting so hormonal," you can say, "Aren't we all?"

Take a look at the fun little roller coaster on the graph of your menstrual cycle hormones:

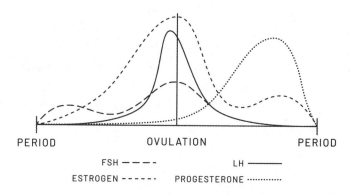

Clearly, your hormones are in constant ebb and flow, and each fluctuation leads to another. It's not as complicated as it may first look.

Technically, a "cycle" by definition has no single beginning and end. But you know what's an easy, visible time to identify where you are in the cycle?

BOOM! You get your period. Doesn't matter whether you like it or not, because big things are happening. Once you start your period, your hormones plummet to their lowest levels of the cycle.

But your body doesn't wait in a low-hormone state for long. **Follicle-stimulating hormone** (her friends call her FSH) comes out to play just days after your period begins.

Your brain's pituitary gland releases FSH. It flows through the bloodstream to the ovaries to tell them to start growing follicles. As those follicles grow, they release the hormone **estrogen**.

I imagine estrogen as your party hormone! As her level increases after your period and peaks at ovulation, she makes you feel good—social, bubbly, confident, like you can do all the things—while keeping your skin, bones, and heart healthy.

Estrogen grows the endometrium and makes your cervical fluid turn into a consistency that supports fertility by helping sperm survive. (Because remember, evolution wants you to get pregnant, even if *you* don't.)

As your estrogen peaks, your testosterone does, too. Then, right before ovulation, your brain's hypothalamus releases a huge surge of **luteinizing hormone** (that's LH for short). LH triggers the most dominant follicle to release the chosen egg of that cycle.

And *that's* ovulation, the main event of your cycle! The special egg tumbles into your pelvic cavity, and the **fimbria**—or little arms—of the fallopian tubes sweep it into a tube, where it may or may not get fertilized by a sperm.

Right after ovulation, estrogen dips way down. This is when **progesterone**, your chill-out hormone, kicks in and becomes the key hormone player. When you have healthy progesterone levels, you keep cool, calm, and collected. Progesterone mellows you out and keeps your uterus healthy by thickening the endometrium, just in case you could be pregnant. (Got imbalanced progesterone levels? Hello, PMS.)

Side note: You might be wondering what happens to the follicle that released the egg. This is wild. The follicle collapses into itself and morphs into a temporary mini organ called the **corpus luteum**, Latin for "yellow body." The corpus luteum is what produces progesterone. And, if you do get pregnant that cycle, the corpus luteum actually turns into the placenta!

Your body will continue to produce progesterone into pregnancy, but if you don't conceive that cycle, the corpus luteum will produce progesterone for about 10 to 16 days, and then it'll disintegrate.

Once it disintegrates, your hormone levels plummet, and BOOM! Another period begins. Rinse and repeat, over and over for most of your reproductive years.

THE GIST OF IT

Alright, alright, if you want to skip the nitty gritty, here's an acronym to help you remember how your hormones flow throughout the cycle: FELOP.

❀ **F:** FSH rises
❀ **E:** Estrogen rises

- ❀ **L:** LH skyrockets
- ❀ **O:** Ovulation occurs
- ❀ **P:** Progesterone kicks in

FELOP describes your hormonal fluctuations and gives you a backdrop to learn the four phases of the menstrual cycle: the foundation of cycle syncing.

THE FOUR PHASES

OVULATION: THE CYCLE'S DIVIDING LINE

Biologically speaking, the menstrual cycle consists of two distinct phases, divided by the moment of ovulation. The follicular phase lasts from the start of a period leading up to the moment of ovulation (it's named after those follicles growing eggs). The luteal phase lasts from the moment of ovulation until the start of the next period (named after the corpus luteum).

But practically and experientially speaking, your period and ovulation are such big events that they produce their own symptoms and "special effects."

This means you can divide the whole cycle into four phases:

- ❀ The menstrual phase (days around period)
- ❀ The follicular phase (days between end of period and leading up to ovulation)
- ❀ The ovulatory phase (days around ovulation)
- ❀ The luteal phase (days after ovulation and leading up to the next period)

HOW TO TELL WHEN YOU'RE OVULATING

The best way to track ovulation and other health data is to chart your cycles (an incredible topic for another book; many people start by reading *Taking Charge of Your Fertility* by Toni Weschler). People who use **fertility awareness**—whether for birth control, to conceive, or to track health—create a chart for each cycle displaying the data of their fertility signs.

Without getting deep into fertility awareness, here are a few signs that you may be approaching ovulation:

- ❀ Keep an eye out for cervical fluid. This is the white or clear stuff that you see on your underwear or in the toilet. It's what helps sperm survive and swim, and it helps prevent infection in our own bodies. As you approach ovulation, you'll notice that your cervical fluid turns from thick, white, and sticky to clear, stretchy, and wet; in fact, it often looks like egg whites.

Then, after ovulation, the fluid reverts back to thick, tacky, and opaque—no more egg white quality.

❀ You might get a bit of red or pink ovulation spotting or a day or two of ovulation pain.

❀ Many menstruators notice increased energy, libido, extroversion, and confidence.

❀ Luteinizing hormone test strips can give you a clue that ovulation might be close to happening, and progesterone test strips can let you know after the fact that ovulation occurred.

If you're not practicing fertility awareness and charting cycles, you can still get a good idea of when you're ovulating. Then, you can build your cycle syncing plans around that knowledge!

COUNTING CYCLE DAYS

Each day of the cycle gets a number to name it. "Cycle Day 1" is always the first day of your period. That means full-flow, true period—not just spotting.

The next day would be "Cycle Day 2," and so on. Many people with regular cycles ovulate around Cycle Days 12 to 16, but that's certainly not the case for everyone.

Just like it's false that everyone ovulates on Cycle Day 14, it's also a myth that most menstruators have 28 day cycles. The average can be anywhere from 25- to 35-day cycles for regular menstruators. Most hormonal birth control is designed to keep you close to 28 days, but most people don't operate that way.

Next time you start your period, call it Cycle Day 1. Keep counting until you get to the next period, which will be the next Cycle Day 1. How high did you count before the next period? That was the length of that cycle.

HOW HORMONAL BIRTH CONTROL CHANGES YOUR CYCLE

Hormonal birth control works by suppressing your natural hormones (and so, your whole cycle) in order to prevent ovulation (how you get pregnant). That means you don't get the roller coaster flow of hormones shown in the last diagram. Instead, the synthetic hormones from hormonal birth control give you a flat line. In the sugar pill week, the sudden withdrawal of those drugs triggers a "withdrawal bleed," which isn't a true period. In order to have a true period, you must ovulate roughly a couple weeks before it.

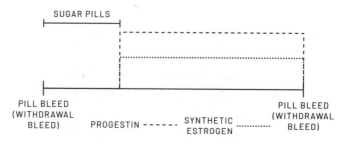

MEDICATED CYCLE
WHILE USING HORMONAL BIRTH CONTROL

SUGAR PILLS

PILL BLEED
(WITHDRAWAL
BLEED)

PROGESTIN ‑ ‑ ‑ ‑ ‑

SYNTHETIC
ESTROGEN

PILL BLEED
(WITHDRAWAL
BLEED)

If, for whatever reason, you make an informed choice to use hormonal birth control, you can still practice cycle syncing. Some people still feel the four seasons as outlined in The Four Seasons (below), even on the pill or IUD. If you don't feel the fluctuations so obviously, then later on we'll cover how to live cyclically without a true menstrual cycle.

HOW CYCLE SYNCING FITS INTO ALL THIS

Have you ever noticed how some weeks you feel like a great speaker and communicator, like the words just come to you? But then, a week later, you'd rather not see—let alone talk—to anyone? Or maybe you feel super strong on your runs for a couple weeks but sluggish leading into your period. You might even love your job half the month and hate it the rest!

You can work with all of that by creatively timing the way you move, eat, work, and play with those four cycle phases we just covered. Your hormone levels are different in each phase, so life can look different from phase to phase. Your cycle is like an almanac to guide you through your inner climate during the coming weeks and months.

THE FOUR SEASONS

Imagine the four seasons of nature. Each season is distinct, yet each blends seamlessly into the next. We can't have one without the other three. Your cycle phases are the same way. And, in fact, those phases align quite nicely with nature's seasons!

You're probably already thinking about your favorite season. I get it—for most of my life, I saw summer as the *best* time, and I dreaded winter. And I saw this in my cycles, too. When I committed to cyclical living, I finally began to discover the incredible benefits of *all four seasons*, both those in my body and those on Earth. Why bother dreading half your cycle, or half the year? I don't know about you, but I want to adore my *entire* life.

Nature designed your menstrual cycle to support evolutionary processes—in other words, life! Nature inherently fluctuates in a sustainable way to make life happen, and you are a natural being. You were born to endure seasons.

How can we be more like nature? Creating more than we take. Giving more than draining. Balancing times of "on" and "off." Waxing and waning like the moon. Rising and falling like the tides. Rising and setting like the sun. Your cycle's seasons allow that to happen in a way that feels healthy and sustainable.

Fighting against that biology is a waste of energy and can even be destructive. Becoming aware of your menstrual cycle helps you move from destruction to creation and growth: of goals, of accomplishments, of your truest self. We're taught only to listen to the mind and ego, but if you're anything like me and want to live a big life, you'll feel more fulfilled if you learn to listen to your body and its seasons, too.

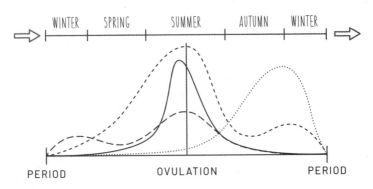

HOW TO KNOW WHICH SEASON YOU'RE IN

Remember the four phases: menstrual, follicular, ovulatory, and luteal? These each line up with an inner season, or a period of time in which you feel, think, and act in a different way based on your internal environment. Imagine the changing energy of each of Earth's seasons; your body experiences those shifts throughout a menstrual cycle, and we'll dig into how that manifests in the coming chapters.

THE CYCLE SYNCING HANDBOOK

For many people, the inner seasons look similar to this:

❀ **Inner winter:** the menstrual phase (days around period)

❀ **Inner spring:** the follicular phase (days between end of period and leading up to ovulation)

❀ **Inner summer:** the ovulatory phase (days around ovulation)

❀ **Inner autumn:** the luteal phase (days after ovulation and leading up to the next period)

Please note: This can vary greatly by individual! If you find after reading the seasons' chapters that your inner seasons line up with different phases of the cycle, by all means, go with that framework.

Here's an example. I personally have an average of a 26-day cycle (26 days from the start of one period to the start of the next).

My unique seasons typically look like this:

❀ My inner winter starts around Cycle Day 24 (before my period arrives), and starts transitioning to spring around Cycle Day 4 (after most of my period and bleeding).

❀ My inner spring transitions to inner summer around days 10 to 11.

❀ My inner summer transitions to inner autumn around days 17 to 18.

❀ My inner autumn transitions to winter around day 24 again, and the cycle repeats.

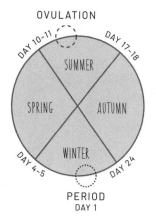

ANGIE'S 26-DAY
CYCLE WITH SEASONS

OVULATION

DAY 10-11 · DAY 17-18

SUMMER

SPRING · AUTUMN

DAY 4-5 · WINTER · DAY 24

PERIOD
DAY 1

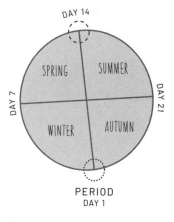

A FRIEND'S 28-DAY
CYCLE WITH SEASONS

DAY 14

SPRING · SUMMER

DAY 7 · DAY 21

WINTER · AUTUMN

PERIOD
DAY 1

Notice that there are overlapping days of transition, and my winter starts a couple of days before my friend's period begins. We experience seasons differently. Your own seasons may line up differently from both these examples. Track yours to see how they look! We'll get into transition days, as well as when your seasons are different lengths from each other, toward the end of this book.

As we dive into each phase, or each season, please remember that there are no strict rules—your lived experience trumps any framework. The key is tracking your cycles to find out how your mind and body respond to each season, then strategize your life around them as best as you can. Fighting nature always makes life harder; you can't change the weather, but you can prepare for it and still enjoy the day.

START NOTICING YOUR OWN SEASONS

Not everybody experiences the inner seasons in the same way. Some people feel most at home in inner autumn, while others love inner summer. Some people love the release of inner winter, while others have period symptoms that hold them back from enjoying it. Some people might even have past trauma or parts of their personality that make the visibility of inner spring difficult to handle.

In order to flow with the seasons, you need to figure out your own unique, seasonal characteristics and transitions. Here's a template you can start using today, as soon as you identify which Cycle Day it is. Use the Inner Season Tracker to take notes for a few cycles to determine the patterns in your own cyclical experience. Every day this cycle, check in with yourself and write simple (or thorough!) notes on how you feel physically, mentally, emotionally, and overall. Even one word is a great start! In just a few cycles, you'll be able to plan what season you'll be in weeks in advance, and be able to predict your mood, energy, and interests.

YOUR INNER SEASON TRACKER

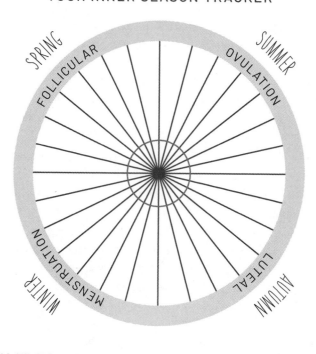

TRACK IT TO HACK IT

Love data? You might add notes about specific facets of wellness to your tracker, an app, or some record you create for yourself. Note the Cycle Day when you observe and collect your data so that you can identify cyclical patterns around it:

❀ Sleep (length, quality, bedtime, fatigue)

❀ Energy (physical, creative, interpersonal)

❀ Mood (self-esteem, libido, socialness, anxiety)

❀ Appetite (hunger, cravings, aversions)

❀ Data from devices (resting heart rate)

❀ Symptoms (bloating, skin issues, digestion)

❀ Fertility signs (cervical fluid, basal body temperature, cervical position)

❀ Any other data that you find interesting to track

You can record observations in these areas as written notes in your tracker. Or, maybe you create coded symbols on an app or in your phone notes, with certain emojis indicating certain symptoms or other data. For example, a cookie emoji can symbolize sweet cravings, or a lightning bolt emoji can represent a high-energy day. Whether you choose to use paper or a digital version, the priority is finding a clear way to note the "what" (symptom/observation) and the "when" (Cycle Days) in a way that makes it easy to compare one cycle to another.

DIGGING INTO EACH SEASON

In the chapters to follow, you'll dive into the powers and challenges of your four inner seasons. You'll find themes, self-care activities, and journaling prompts for each season, but remember the three pillars of cycle syncing:

※ **Manage your energy, not your time:** If you're like most of us, you feel the urge to "do it all," all the time. It can be hard to shake off those old urges and habits. Remind yourself that each season sets itself up for the next one, bringing a whole different energy that's suited to different tasks.

※ **Play over perfection:** No need to follow seasonal suggestions to a T. Use them as a starting point to experiment and brainstorm what feels best to you. Adding how you honored your inner season into your Inner Season Tracker can help you keep note of what experiments went well.

※ **Your experience above all:** If your ovulatory phase feels more like inner winter than your menstrual phase does, more power to you. Every menstruator is different, so align the seasons with what works for you. Use the Inner Season Tracker to find your own patterns!

SUMMARY

Your menstrual cycle isn't a mystery; it's a cyclical pattern that you can predict and get to know intimately. Without this process, we wouldn't all be here, living our lives. It's a crucial cycle in the human body, and we can learn to be proud of it instead of ashamed.

And, we can learn to take advantage of it through what you came here for: cycle syncing.

If you skipped over all the science, read at least this:

※ Every cycle, your body prepares for a potential pregnancy by releasing an egg. If pregnancy does not occur, you get your period, which is the shedding of your uterine lining.

※ To make this process happen, there are four phases of hormone levels that you experience throughout a single menstrual cycle.

THE CYCLE SYNCING HANDBOOK

✺ Each phase aligns with an inner season that influences how you think, feel, act, and perform.

✺ The menstrual phase is inner winter, the follicular phase is inner spring, the ovulatory phase is inner summer, and the luteal phase is inner autumn.

✺ Each season is equally important and leads perfectly into the next, so you experience four different inner seasons over the course of a cycle.

✺ You *can* do anything at any time. But why not try scheduling your tasks and goals for when they'll come even easier to you?

CHAPTER 2

INNER WINTER

● ● ●

How do you imagine the energy of winter?

As winter falls, the planet gets darker, quieter, and slower. Animals hibernate peacefully, the garden soil rests undisturbed, and the starry skies get especially clear. It's as if every living thing is subtly reenergizing for the months ahead—and guess what? So are you.

Welcome to inner winter, overlapping with your menstrual phase, or the time around and during your period.

THE MENSTRUAL PHASE

During your period, estrogen and progesterone levels drop to their lowest of the entire menstrual cycle. Your body has realized that it is indeed not pregnant, so it sheds your uterine lining to give the womb another chance at pregnancy later on in this cycle (whether or not that's what you want!).

Research shows that brain communication between its hemispheres is greatest during menstruation; there are more synaptic connections between the left (analytical) and right (emotional) sides of the brain.[2] This makes your period an opportune time to reflect on your past and decide what you really desire going forward.

HOW YOU KNOW YOU'RE ENTERING INNER WINTER

❀ It feels like premenstrual tension (finally!) eases away.

❀ It could feel like you're going to bleed soon, or your bleed actually starts.

. . . .
2 Stephanie Cacioppo et. al, "Hemispheric Specialization Varies with EEG Brain Resting States and Phase of Menstrual Cycle," *Plos One* 8, no. 4 (2013): e63196, https://www.ncbi.nlm.nih.gov/pmc/articles/PMC3640095.

❀ You may experience menstrual cramps.

❀ You may feel emotionally ready to let go, or notice a deep inward focus. You might even feel like you're entering a dreamlike, spacey state.

❀ Basal body temperature, or your body's core resting temperature, drops. People who practice fertility awareness often record their lowest temperatures of the night. This core temperature rises after ovulation and remains elevated until around the start of the next cycle.

A BUILT-IN REMINDER TO REST

The menstrual phase is the part of your cycle that reminds you to slow down and rest every once in a while, like those hibernating animals. You might crave relaxation and alone time more than you normally would.

High-performing people often struggle with this phase, since slowing down can seem counterproductive. But think of a garden: Nothing blooms all year round. The winter season is necessary to ensure growth in the warmer months. Farmers use the winter before a busy spring to fix equipment, plan, and prepare. Every part of the cycle is necessary. In order to bloom, you need to rest, as well. Let your period be your nudge to ease off temporarily.

Take one of my favorite reminders: even though you *can* do it all, you don't *have* to.

YOU CAN DO ANYTHING ON YOUR PERIOD, AS LONG AS YOU WANT TO

In the period world, I've noticed a false dichotomy: Some people say, "Rest is the only way for your period! Lie on the couch and chill for a few days." Meanwhile, others follow the "Anything you can do, I can do while bleeding" ethos, and claim that your period shouldn't hold you back from *anything*. Neither side is right, and neither is wrong.

You can do *anything you want to* on your period; I'm not saying that a period is a time to remove yourself from the world, your responsibilities, and the things you enjoy! Nature wouldn't design you to be on bed rest for a fifth to a quarter of the year. You are most certainly *not* a weaker version of yourself while bleeding.

Many menstruators do find that rest comes most naturally at this time, and a bleed is a reminder that you can *choose* to rest if you need or want to. The bonus? Rest allows you to build up energy reserves for the inner spring and inner summer ahead.

So, do you feel like playing in the big game on Cycle Day 1? Awesome, have fun! Know in your gut you'd rather stay at home in the bath? You do you. Want to host a party during your period? Yay! Want to lie in a cocoon instead? Go for it.

It's not about whether you should or shouldn't do things on your period. It's about asking yourself every day, "What do I truly want and need?" Then, make your decisions from an empowered place, not an arbitrary rule.

SETTING UP THE REST OF YOUR CYCLE FOR SUCCESS

Remember, your menstrual phase, or inner winter, sets the scene for the rest of the cycle. Give yourself the restoration you need now so that you can kick butt harnessing the strengths of the other three seasons.

If you don't give yourself this periodic down time, it's possible that you'll struggle to develop the powers of inner spring, feel burned out later on in the month, or exacerbate period symptoms. In fact, those very symptoms may be asking you to slow down temporarily.

Of course, slowing down a bit can open up more time to reflect on how the following weeks can get you closer to your dream life. If you allow it, inner winter is a fantastic time to take stock of where you're currently at and what steps you may take in the near future to bring your dreams closer to reality.

POWERS OF INNER WINTER

INTUITION AND SELF-CONNECTION

We're inundated with external opinions, pressures, and ideas almost every day. Your inner winter dims all that noise a bit, fading external cues so that you can focus more on your internal cues. This season allows you to reset your compass to point toward where *you* want to go, without external voices getting in the way.

You'll be more intuitive so you can decide what you need to let go of and what you want to give attention to in the coming weeks. Feeling any emotions that arise here will help point you in the right direction. The things that bother you during your period are the things that bother you the rest of your cycle, too—you'll just finally notice them during your period. Stillness reveals the truth.

STILLNESS

Of all the seasons, inner winter is the easiest one in which to allow yourself to simply be. You'll be more drawn to solitude and quiet spaces, giving you the stillness you need to reconnect with what you most need and desire in life.

Even just sitting with an idea and letting it roll around in your head without an agenda can pay off later on. It's like how many people get "shower ideas," jolts of inspiration that seem to randomly pop in their head when they relax in the shower. The relative stillness of your period lends itself to "period ideas."

AWARENESS

Inner winter brings about a sixth sense of sorts. There are times where you might go back and forth over a decision for weeks and then when you get your period, you know exactly what to do. These revelations can bring needed clarity and greater awareness about your role, your purpose, and the life you want to live.

Inner winter also brings about strong awareness of the five senses. The way you sense things can be elevated at this time, which is why it can be helpful to focus on pleasurable sensations (even a soft blanket can feel cozier now).

RESTORATION AND HEALING

Inner winter is an ideal time to practice letting things go. We build up "stuff" all cycle, whether it be feelings, tension, fears, anxieties, struggles, or thoughts. Inner winter is the opportunity to release all of that so you can truly relax and rejuvenate both your mind and your body.

If you allow for the time and space, this is the most efficient season to soothe your nervous system, calm down, and let go of tension. Hopefully, your previous inner autumn season afforded you the space in inner winter to nourish and rejuvenate yourself.

ACCEPTANCE AND FORGIVENESS

Start asking yourself, "Can I just let this be?" Imagine the relief that comes from releasing pent-up feelings and harmful thoughts. Sometimes, the best way forward is simply to accept them (and even let them go). This is your chance to let things sit without trying to change them. You may find it's easier to let go of resentment, past arguments, and ruminating thoughts in your head.

You can forgive yourself and others more easily. After all, it's a fresh beginning with so many good times ahead.

Your winter is your time just to let things be what they are, just like there are no seeds to plant and no fruits to harvest. By clearing out the old, you allow new opportunities to come in, like the golden sunflowers down the road.

CHALLENGES OF INNER WINTER

SOCIETAL PRESSURES

In our busy society, we're expected to be 100 percent "on," 100 percent of the time. So, of course, it can be difficult to slow down! Even if your body and brain are begging you to take a pause, the nagging voices in your head won't allow it when there's "so much to do." They whisper constant distractions of what you *should* be doing, which takes away from your true rest and inner winter powers.

These voices can make it hard to stay present and slow down. But slowing down isn't a full stop. As you begin to practice cycle syncing, can you identify how you can slow down by just 10 percent? Especially if you know that not allowing for any rest here will decrease the productivity of the inner spring and inner summer to come? Maybe you can let the house be a tiny bit messier than usual, have the teenager next door walk the dog, or order takeout for dinner instead of cooking it yourself. What small tasks can you take off your plate for a few days?

GUILT

When you take time off from responsibilities or take a step back, even temporarily, it's easy to feel guilty for not "doing it all" or for saying no to favors. But what if you tried easing back, and the world didn't fall apart?

You could take it even further, if easing up by 10 percent feels good. The idea of "doing nothing" is hard to fathom; we all have responsibilities! But what would happen if you took a half day simply to do nothing "useful" or "productive"? If that's too scary, what about 30 minutes? Could you try just 10 minutes a day during inner winter? Try it, and you'll work through the guilt that we shouldn't have to feel, anyway.

PERIOD PROBLEMS

If you have rough period symptoms, I feel you. Dealing with pain can make it extremely difficult to embrace inner winter—not to mention, quality of life suffers with extreme symptoms.

THE CYCLE SYNCING HANDBOOK

If you haven't gotten medical care for your period problems yet, start tracking data now. When do you experience symptoms? What do they feel like? What do signs look like? How much do you bleed, and when, and what color? You can start noting this data on your Inner Season Tracker from Chapter X.

Keep in mind that your period itself isn't the problem; its negative symptoms are signs that there's an issue with a system in your body. Period problems are common, but that doesn't mean they're normal. The more data you can collect around your symptoms, the more information you can give a medical care provider to narrow down causes.

A healthy period comes every 25 to 35 days, lasts 3 to7 days, is a bright cranberry red in color, and has a slightly thick texture without big clots. When should you check with a doctor? I recommend doing so if you experience bleeding over 80 milliliters over one period (that's soaking through over 16 regular pads or tampons), bleed for only one to two days or over seven days, have less than 25 days between the start of one period and the start of the next, have unpredictable periods, struggle with premenstrual symptoms, have more than mild cramping or pain, or any other symptoms that significantly interfere with your life.

SELF-CARE AND RITUALS
TO TRY THIS CYCLE

How can you nurture those cozy inner winter vibes in this season? Even if you can only squeeze in 20 minutes of intentional rest a day, use that time to slow down and focus on only yourself. This is *purposeful* rest—it allows you to work hard the rest of your cycle!

Take a look at the ideas below and see what sounds appealing to you in this season. Can you commit to incorporating one to three next inner winter?

HOW YOU CAN BEGIN TO EMBRACE INNER WINTER

❀ Create a bite-size mini "hibernation" each inner winter day, even if it's just a short nap.

❀ On Cycle Day 1, write out the rest of your Cycle Days on your calendar so you can glance at your calendar and predict how you'll feel each week.

❀ Block out a day (or days) in advance on your calendar with a symbol representing inner winter, so you remember to plan fewer engagements for those times.

- Pick one area of life to take a bit of time off from. Perhaps that's work, traveling, household chores, home renovations, blogging, social plans, cooking, or volunteering. What's one responsibility that won't completely fall apart if you pulled back for a few days?
- Take a few days off social media.
- Take a work-from-home day if you usually work outside the home.
- Organize a "kid swap" with a friend so you can watch each other's kids while one is experiencing their inner winter.
- Catch up on those little things you've been eyeing: watch a new show, listen to a favorite podcast, or look into something that's piquing your curiosity.
- Light some candles, snuggle with a soft blanket, and go to bed early.
- Get your nails done or book a massage.
- Sit outside in a peaceful, natural space for lunch.
- Schedule a 5- to 10-minute meditation or breathwork session before opening your laptop.
- Start the book you've been wanting to read.
- Go to a yin yoga class.
- Create a vision board for the upcoming cycle or for your life.
- Curate a relaxing playlist.
- Use red sheets or towels to remind you of your inner winter (and possibly prevent stains, which happen!).
- Give yourself a gift every inner winter. Create a self-care box reserved just for during your period. It may have special underwear, tea, candles, your favorite chocolate, something cozy to wear, intention cards, or anything that brings you a bit of joy and comfort during that time.
- Set an intention or goal for the coming cycle, and keep a journal to track your energy trends throughout the cycle.
- Take a deep look at the coming month's goals and plans. Meditate, visualize, or journal about the weeks ahead and set benchmarks you'd like to meet toward your goals. Imagine what you'd love to happen in this cycle, determine what your focal priorities will be, and consider how you'd like to feel between now and your next period. Using all of that, set an intention for the cycle.

THE CYCLE SYNCING HANDBOOK

❀ Get closure from the *past* cycle by adding an element of reflection to every inner winter season. That might be journaling, reviewing your accomplishments, or organizing your photos.

JOURNAL PROMPTS FOR INNER WINTER

This season is perfect for free-flow writing and dreaming. If you don't feel like writing, you can create another type of art to represent the start of a new cycle.

❀ What is your intention for this cycle?

❀ List what you have been grateful for recently.

❀ What clarity do you seek?

❀ What no longer serves you? Can you release it?

❀ Write three pages. Just let anything come out.

❀ What is something you love about yourself?

❀ Is there anything that requires more of your attention?

· ·

TRY IT: A TINY TWEAK FOR THE BUSY MENSTRUATOR

Dedicate 15 minutes per day of your inner winter to doing something that feels restorative to you, whether that's listening to music while stretching, a reflection session, looking at a beautiful coffee table book, watching part of your favorite show, or anything else that can give you a microburst of joy.

· ·

· ·

TRY IT: A BOLD MOVE FOR THE DEVOTED CYCLE SYNCER

Every cycle, take one entire day—perhaps the first day of your period—to fully devote to yourself and to *whatever* feels good. Schedule no meetings, save the deep work for another day, and dress comfortably. Then, spend your day (or allotted hours) doing and being without any goal of "productivity." Remember, it's just one day per cycle. You won't fall behind (it's a part of the process!), and it'll leave you refreshed and feeling ready to move forward powerfully.

I often use this time as a "life admin" catch-up day; it's not very glamorous, but I get recharged by the solo time spent doing mundane tasks I *have* to do but that can be batched for a lazy day while listening to music with my laptop on the couch. If I simply remove the pressure of being productive and instead allow whatever happens to happen, I'm often surprised at what tasks I finish while still feeling rested and slow paced.

When I start a new habit or even a new, big project, I love to list out three reasons why I'm committing to it. I literally write them down so I can revisit them when motivation starts to wane. How will this habit help future you? Jot it down!

. . . .

INNER WINTER'S LIFE LESSON: LIVING BY YOUR VALUES

Although inner winter can be a very intuitive time, our society often makes it difficult to follow our intuition! Sometimes, you might *think* you know what to do, but the what-ifs pop into your brain and cloud your options even more.

When this happens to me, I return to my core values. Values are the concepts or feelings that you hold most important in life, the experiences that make you feel most fulfilled. They subconsciously and consciously drive you to act and behave in certain ways, based on what motivates you in life. Often, they're what cause you to make decisions toward fulfillment and the life you want to live (if you follow them).

As a former perfectionist, I struggled with saying no to opportunities, even if they weren't a great fit for me at that time. Work opportunities, social activities, volunteer positions—I figure I *could* do them all, so why not? The wonderful life coach Melanie McCloskey, knowing my love for hiking and mountaineering, gently pointed out to me, "Be mindful about climbing the wrong mountains just because you love to climb."

It hit me: so many past opportunities weren't fulfilling to me because they didn't align with my core values. I always said yes because I loved the feeling of achievement, even if those achievements weren't meaningful in the long term. Although those opportunities were all mountains on the horizon, they weren't the right mountains for me to climb!

THE CYCLE SYNCING HANDBOOK

Now, when I'm faced with an opportunity, decision, or even the broad question "What's next?," I sit and consider my values. In particular, I need to honor the values of health, freedom, exploration, growth, and empowerment (as defined by me) in order to feel like I'm living my best life. If a "mountain" doesn't align with those top core values, I understand that my response to climb it might be a no or a maybe someday instead of an obligatory yes.

I find that inner winter is an excellent time to revisit my values, especially if I'm struggling to connect with or follow my intuition. When you're setting goals or intentions for your cycle, you can consider your core values to be your North Star. Does that goal or intention align with what you hold most important in life? Is this cycle the cycle to focus on it? Or are you climbing the wrong mountain just because you love to climb?

TAKE IT FURTHER: MAKING BIG DECISIONS ON YOUR PERIOD

I like to wait to make big decisions (when time allows) until after a full cycle, including a full inner winter. If you're facing a big life choice, you can use inner spring to research options, inner summer to discuss it with others, inner autumn to reflect heavily on the truth, and inner winter to come to your decision intuitively.

In fact, I waited to decide on whether or not to write this book until I experienced an entire cycle. The clarity I reached on my period—yes, I *did* truly want to write this book!—was what I needed to make a confident, fully informed choice on something that would take an immense amount of effort and time.

WHAT FELLOW MENSTRUATORS SAY

❀ "I've finally started to listen to my body, and my quality of life has been elevated. I no longer fight against my body's needs. Now my inner winter feels calm and restorative. I am able to lean into the rest and understand what my body needs to prepare for the rest of my seasons." —Paige

❀ "There's a relief that comes when my period arrives, and I always have the thought, 'Oohhh, so that's why I've been feeling so blah.'" —Dani

❋ "I actually feel like a freaking superhero while bleeding. It's like I'm most at one with my wild self, but also like a secret nobody else gets to know."
—Lynn

•   •   •

INNER WINTER ALMANAC WORKSHEET

Use this worksheet to get to know *your* inner winter. Make a photocopy so you can return to it each cycle for the next few months.

1. Imagine Earth's season of winter. What words come to mind when you think about the energy behind wintertime?

_____

2. Considering the words you just wrote, what are some tiny ways you could enhance that energy in your everyday life?

_____

_____

_____

3. What Cycle Days do you notice that you're in your inner winter? (Remember, Cycle Day 1 is the first day of your full flow period.)

_____

4. Next time you find yourself in inner winter, note any obstacles that show up here:

_____

_____

_____

_____

_____

5. Jot down any personal strengths you notice that come out during inner winter:

----

6. While you're in your inner winter, brain dump all the things that sound appealing and fulfilling in this part of your cycle:

Come back to this worksheet each inner winter for a few cycles, and you'll start to paint a very clear picture of what the season looks like for *you*.

●　　●　　●

TRANSITIONING TO INNER SPRING

The transition from inner winter to inner spring typically occurs toward the end of your period, or after it finishes. Of course, timing is different for everyone. You might have a short period, with inner winter lasting days after bleeding ends. You might have started inner winter before your period, and are now starting inner spring while still bleeding. Notice *your* patterns!

As you transition, you might feel lighter emotionally, physically, and energetically. You'll start to feel mentally clear and focused, with a desire to get out into the world again.

The sudden visibility of spring can be jarring, if you're not mindful. Flowers can't go from seed to full bloom immediately; they need to sprout first, poking stems above the dirt and slowly growing taller. As you enter inner spring, think of yourself as the sprout. Emerging too quickly from the ground could feel blinding at first.

SUMMARY

Before they start to live more cyclically, many menstruators dread their periods. They often try to push through discomfort, ruminate in inner winter's challenges, and get frustrated that they're not blooming in the way a garden would in summertime.

But the reality is that without the rest, restoration, and slowness of inner winter, the other seasons wouldn't have their time to shine. In fact, the inherent qualities of inner winter can be extremely powerful ways to allow you to shine, as well!

If you find inner winter a pleasant season for you, start going a bit deeper. Consider your long-term dreams and how inner winter's powers can help you get there.

If inner winter is still a challenge for you, pick one self-care idea from this chapter to apply next period. Then, with each passing period, add one more. They don't need to be huge feats; it's about adding subtle tools to increase joy in your everyday life.

CHAPTER 3

INNER SPRING

· · ·

When you envision the energy behind spring, what words come to mind?

When spring arrives, there's a buzz to the world. The burst of liveliness after a winter slumber is energizing. Birds chirp early in the morning and sprouts poke through the ground to greet the sun. The planet is reawakening, and you might feel the same way! This is inner spring, which coincides with the follicular phase, or the time after your period and leading up toward ovulation.

THE FOLLICULAR PHASE

As your inner winter and period end, you enter your follicular phase, which is just like spring.

Biologically, your ovaries are back at work trying to get egg follicles to develop and your uterine lining starts rebuilding. From an evolutionary lens, your biology wants you to start socializing again, in hopes that you'll find a potential mate. Physically and mentally, you start feeling more energetic and like you want to reconnect with the world.

As your period ends, you might feel the urge to jump right back into a busy, fast-paced life, but try to ease into this inner spring so you don't burn out. You may have more energy and have a to-do list to complete, but continue to be gentle with yourself. You can harness this energy for the rest of your cycle if you don't overdo it right away. Your garden doesn't jump straight to full bloom—you need to plan out and tend to the garden first.

HOW YOU KNOW YOU'RE ENTERING INNER SPRING

❀ You feel a spark within yourself that excites you.

❀ You feel a sense of "reawakening" after the lower energy of your period.

❀ You might feel more motivated, social, and confident.

❀ You may notice an increase in sexual desire.

❀ Your period ends, or you notice an increase in cervical mucus and/or vaginal lubrication.

STRATEGIZING YOUR LIFE

If you're a list maker, planner, or sticky note jotter, you'll likely love spring. Just like plants sprouting out of the earth after winter, the ideas and opportunities sprout all around you! Hopefully, you crafted a vision in your inner winter, and spring is the time to strategize.

Before you get down to work, take a second to reflect: "What exactly am I growing this cycle?" Is there a budding project at work? A new relationship? A change in habits you're itching to implement? Is it a side business idea, a health issue you're finally addressing, a home renovation, a new website? Whatever you could be growing, does it fulfill the intentions you set in winter?

Sometimes, the amount of growth inherent in spring can feel overwhelming, like you exited the period hibernation cave and have no idea which colorful path to start down. Often, the first step to strategizing is a brain dump. List out *all* the potential paths, ideas, and goals you could work toward this cycle. Then, cut it down. What is the *main* goal you'd like to work on this cycle? (Remember, you'll have plenty more cycles–pick what makes sense today!)

Then, dig into planning. What are the very first steps to that goal? (The smaller, the better.) What will the bigger steps be (that perhaps you could take in inner summer)? Who's on your team whom you could ask for support? How will you know you've achieved the goal, and what will it feel like?

Researching and planning are key to the creative process. No matter what you're "growing" in your life, take time in inner spring to get strategic.

PROTOTYPING IDEAS

Before you get carried away with an exciting direction (look at that thing sprout!), consider creating a prototype. A prototype is a rudimentary model of something that will someday be bigger and more complex. This simple, starter version of an idea will lay the foundation for a future product after feedback and more iterations.

In other words, it's an easy example of your idea that you don't need to feel too attached to, since it doesn't take much time to create! In fact, they say that if you're not at least a little embarrassed by your first version of something, then you probably waited too long to put it out there.

Got an idea for an event series in town? Want to start offering design services online? Have a great idea for the best hiking backpack design ever? Whatever your inner spring brain blast is, take a beat to consider what the "minimum viable product" would be, to borrow from business terms. What could you put together *this cycle* that would sufficiently test your idea so you can collect feedback and see if it's worth pursuing further?

I like to ask myself, "What is the smallest step forward I could take now that I could afford to lose from?" *That's* entrepreneurial thinking.

You'll be inspired by *so* many things in your inner spring, but try to keep some of your many ideas to yourself to let them grow and strengthen before you share them with the world. You're not aiming for outcomes or results quite yet—you'll save that for summer and autumn. So pick one main project that inspires you, table the rest, and create a prototype that you can expand on in future cycles, after you let it go through the creative process of *this* cycle.

STARTING NEW HABITS

Inner spring is the optimal time to form new habits. Your motivation is high, you're inspired by new ideas, and you're not afraid to play around and try new things.

Consider your cycle intention. How do you want to feel when you reflect back on this very cycle? What can you do every day, or habitually, in order to end up feeling that way?

The tricky part about habits—what often makes them so hard to stick—is that we tend not to design them intentionally. We ask ourselves, "What do I want?" which usually doesn't have enough inherent motivation to keep the habit.

Instead, we could ask, "What kind of person do I want to be, and what would that kind of person do?"

Instead of "I want to run a 50k," you may ask, "What would an ultramarathoner do? How do they live?" and allow your habits to flow from that. It's hard at first, but separating the outcome from the process can let the magic happen. Focus on the process of becoming the person you want to be rather than solely on an outcome you want.

Try spending time in inner winter asking whom you want to be. Come inner spring, you'll be itching to implement those habits to make you realize that version of yourself!

POWERS OF INNER SPRING

CURIOSITY AND IMAGINATION

Inner spring feels magical; you can sense the potential within you and in the world. There are so many options available to you, and you can explore them since nothing is finalized yet (that's for later in the cycle!). Get curious about what's attracting you, and imagine what a future could look like.

Sign up for a class to learn something totally new. Meet friends of friends. Take a different way to work. Go to a new restaurant. Find ways, big or small, to scratch your curiosity itch and imagine what could be possible. You want to learn, and it'll come easily for you here.

STRATEGY

Okay, so you've got big dreams. But dreams without doing stay dreams. *This* is the time to make a game plan. You're action oriented, rational, logical, and practical in inner spring, so use it to your advantage. This strength is highly valued in our society's workplaces, so lean into it now so that you don't have to force it later on when it comes less naturally to you.

PLAYFULNESS AND SPONTANEITY

Time to let out your inner kid. Remember what it felt like in grade school those first few warm days of the year, when you could finally go outside for recess without a jacket?! Inner winter was a quieter, more serious time. Mix it up and throw some levity and play back into your life in inner spring, just like you did as a kid.

You're less intuitive and more impulsive in this season, so you're drawn to new ideas and experiences. Add novelty wherever you can to lean into the playfulness and spontaneity that you crave! Seek a physical or mental challenge, see a comedy show, try a new, bold outfit. Whatever it is, now's the time to try it out.

FOCUS

Although tons of ideas and opportunities can be inspiring at this time, once you choose where to set your sight, you can really buckle down to focus. Sit down to work with an intentional goal and eliminate outside distractions, and you'll be amazed at what you can get done in a short time. You're primed for deep work at this time, so take advantage. This is your cue to write the outline, set the budget, or rework your website.

You can also *re-focus* on what you've dropped and want to pick back up. What do you need to recommit to? A budget? Cooking for yourself? Checking in with old friends? A training plan?

MOTIVATION

After you've reawakened out of inner winter, you're rejuvenated and refreshed to go after whatever's next. Many people find that they're motivation comes back *strong*, whether it's building confidence, habits, fitness, or a social network.

It's awesome to feel inspired and motivated, but you also need to take action. If you've determined what you truly desire in your inner winter, use the built-in motivation of inner spring to start making progress.

CHALLENGES OF INNER SPRING

SHINY DISTRACTIONS

Ah, the possibilities! All of them sound appealing and doable—so why not do them all? Careful, that thinking is a trap of inner spring's excitement. If you end up being pulled in multiple directions, you may not have enough resources to get after what your inner winter asked you to work on. And then, you could miss out on the coming summer's productivity. And *then*, in inner autumn, you'll feel frustrated that you have nothing to edit and complete!

Use your powers in this phase to strategize and focus on what matters *most*. That doesn't mean you can't get to all the other fun ideas—you might just need to let them breathe for a bit. I like to keep an Inspiration List for all those ideas that I don't want to forget, but also know in my heart it's not the optimal time for. Try it on those days when shiny distractions surround you, but you know you need to commit to your cycle's intention first.

OVEREXPOSURE

With increased confidence and so many great ideas, you may feel the urge to reveal more to the outside world than you're truly ready to. You announce a new business before you sit down to truly plan your vision. You invite folks over for a party in a couple weeks without noticing you'll be in late autumn (and not in a party mood at all). You say "yes" to everything, then soon regret taking on too many commitments.

Think about early spring in an orchard: if there's a late frost, early buds can die, making the rest of the season fruitless. Keep some ideas to yourself a bit longer, until you're further along into a warm weather season and your ideas can be unleashed to others confidently.

JUMPING IN TOO QUICKLY

If your energy starts falling instead of rising through inner spring, you likely either pushed too hard in previous seasons, or you rushed the transition from winter to spring. Just like the planet's seasons, you can't jump from winter to full-on spring overnight! There's a gentle transition as the Earth gets greener, warmer, and more alive; it's not all at once. You might feel an unwelcome, unexpected fatigue creep in if you didn't transition easefully. You took on too much too soon, trying to jump into peak spring energy without allowing a build-up.

Something to consider if you deal with spring fatigue is period-related conditions that affect your energy. Some menstruators with heavy periods struggle with iron deficiency anemia, for example. If you suspect something's up with your period, chat with a doctor and get blood testing so you can fix your energy issues.

SELF-CARE AND RITUALS TO TRY THIS CYCLE

Getting excited? Awesome—but harness that energy intentionally, not just for the sake of *doing*. As you dive into new projects and experiences, keep yourself energized yet grounded with self-care strategies that will set you up for sustainable work and play in the weeks to come.

Consider the list below. Which ideas sound like natural fits for your life? Can you pick one to three to try next inner spring?

HOW YOU CAN BEGIN TO EMBRACE INNER SPRING

❀ Have a "spring clean." Replace the towels and sheets, vacuum the dust, and add some flowers to the table.

❀ Do whatever primping makes you feel good: get your hair, nails, or waxing done.

❀ Try a new-to-you group fitness class or hike a trail you've never seen before.

❀ Grab a few fruits and veggies you don't normally have at home and experiment with new recipes.

❀ Learn anything new: take a short course, read a book on a topic you don't know much about, or listen to a podcast that'll teach you something.

❀ Revisit a previous brain-dump list and see if you're inspired to pick up something you dropped before.

❀ Set time limits on social media. With endless content at your fingertips, you might find yourself scrolling for more and more ideas that take you away from your focus.

❀ Send a message to an old friend or colleague whom you wish you'd stayed in touch with.

❀ Attend a city council or other group meeting to learn about what they do.

❀ Hang out with some kiddos to bring out your imagination.

❀ Treat yourself to some new pens, sticky notes, and stickers that'll add some cheer to your workflow.

❀ Get out your favorite cookbooks and make a shopping list for ingredients for recipes you haven't yet tried.

❀ Wear the fun new outfit.

❀ Volunteer for a day.

JOURNAL PROMPTS FOR INNER SPRING

Moving your newfound energy out of your body and onto something tangible—even just pen and paper—can help get your progress rolling. Accountability is everything. Find a system that will help you integrate this habit for the rest of your cycle. Stick it in your calendar, create an accountability chart to check off each day, or have a trusted friend check in on you.

- ✻ What is a project you'd like to revisit?
- ✻ Is there a relationship you'd like to revitalize?
- ✻ How can you best balance your energy in the coming week?
- ✻ What is overwhelming you? How can you cope?
- ✻ What is a daily source of inspiration for you right now?
- ✻ Describe a time you felt like your most authentic self.
- ✻ What is something that is stirring your curiosity?

TRY IT: A TINY TWEAK FOR THE BUSY MENSTRUATOR

During inner spring, schedule just 20 minutes a day to play or to explore something that's piquing your curiosity. That's it, 20 minutes! You never know where that newfound interest will lead, especially if you don't feed it.

TRY IT: A BOLD MOVE FOR THE DEVOTED CYCLE SYNCER

Start a new, intentional habit! Recall the powers of your inner winter. Where do you have clarity around the need for a new habit? What's the vision you have in implementing a new habit? What kind of person do you want to become as a result of integrating this new habit into your everyday life?

SPRING'S LIFE LESSON: TRUST THE PROCESS

You know how when you're having a bad week of workouts while training for a sports event, and the coach says to "trust the process"? Or you, say, sign a book contract and have no idea how you'll fill up hundreds of pages out of nothing, but you have faith that it'll somehow come together?

Sounds cheesy and esoteric, but trusting the process *works*. Every time I train for an ultramarathon, I find myself on a run wondering, "How the *heck* am I supposed to run 35 miles in a couple months when just these 5 feel long?" Even on my longest training run for 50ks, a 4-hour run, it hits me that that longest run is only about two thirds of the actual race distance. How could that possibly mean I can run the full race?! Deep breath. I remind myself to trust the training process. And I end up finishing the goal race strong.

When you're in the thick of it, the desired end goal may seem impossible. But a complete process sets you up for success, whether it's a well-designed training plan, the creative process, or the menstrual cycle.

Every inner spring, in the depths of doing the work, I wonder, "But *how* is this project going to come to life? Can I just skip ahead? Am I nuts for thinking this will even work?!" I have to remind myself: that experience *is* the process. Spring is just one quarter of the entire cycle; I won't and can't have everything figured out by then. I trust that if I stay on course and follow my strategy, I'll work toward my end goal, even if I can't clearly see it in the distance yet.

The menstrual cycle teaches us that we need to have a balance of making it happen with letting it happen. We need structure and strategy, and we also need room for free flow and surprises. We need to be patient with the process and trust that small steps every day lead to great distances over cycles.

TAKE IT FURTHER: THE 80/20 RULE

Ever heard of the Pareto Principle, also known as the 80/20 Rule? This concept states that 80 percent of your results come from 20 percent of your effort. In other words, 80 percent of what you experience comes from just 20 percent of your habits and actions. If you can nail down the 20 percent of your actions that will best support your goals, you'll feel efficient, fulfilled, and in flow way more often.

The 80/20 Rule can carry over into all areas of your life. What 20 percent of your efforts make the most positive impact on your health? Your home life? Your work and creativity? How can you prioritize those 20 percent of to-dos every day, even if you don't get to the other 80 percent of what you *could* be doing?

Everybody's 20 percent is different, and you can't compare yourself to others. Here's how you can start to identify *your* 20% actions. Let's use work as an example. Grab a pen and paper. On the left side of a sheet, write: "All the Tasks I Have to Do at Work." On the right side, write "Biggest Career Wins So Far." Brain dump answers to write under each column. When you're done, draw lines connecting the wins to the most influential tasks that made it happen. Finally, circle the tasks that have the most connecting lines, the tasks that were responsible for the most wins. Those are your 20 percent.

An entrepreneur might find that most of her customers came from hosting local events, while hardly any came from social media. She can now prioritize events as one of her top 20 percent tasks to grow her business. *And* she now has data to show that she doesn't need to spend much time on social media, since it isn't growing her business much. She can choose to stop social media marketing altogether and reinvest that saved time into events, or she could delegate social media to someone else helping her business.

A blogger might notice that 80 percent of their website traffic comes from just 20 percent of their blog posts. Identifying those top-performing posts allows the blogger to hone in on what people want to read about, informing new posts that drive even more traffic to the blog over time. Plus, the blogger doesn't have to waste time on the 80 percent of posts that *don't* make a significant impact.

What about you? What 20 percent of foods help you feel your healthiest? Stock up on them. What services give you 80 percent of your profit? How can you better focus on those? Which few personal relationships bring you the most joy, and how can you see them more?

In short? Be badass at your 20 percent basics. Ease up on or delegate the rest.

Inspired? Look at cycle syncing through an 80/20 lens: If you cycle sync 20 percent of your life, you'll get 80 percent of the benefits of cyclical living. If you identify your 20 percent of tasks that make the most positive impact on your life, how can you adapt them for each inner season so that you consistently complete them?

WHAT FELLOW
MENSTRUATORS SAY

✸ "I feel I have a lot of new ideas in this phase and want to take action on projects and get things done." —Rachel

THE CYCLE SYNCING HANDBOOK

❀ "Spring is my absolute favorite. I feel more inspired than ever and honestly end up bouncing out of bed in the morning to get to work!" —Precious

❀ "It's kind of jarring for my body. Sometimes I'm not ready to get into action mode and I'd rather stay in winter another day or two." —Tilly

TRANSITIONING TO INNER SUMMER

If you track your cycles, you may notice the transition to summer starts a few days before you ovulate. Your cervical mucus increases, as does your sexual desire. It might not be purely sexual, either—you might feel "turned on" by life itself!

This transition can be like an inner momentum driving you forward. You get progressively more social, energetic, and bold. You start to feel in flow, like you're great at what you do and can't wait to do it more, full of gratitude and positivity. In fact, you might find that opportunities arise out of nowhere to land in your lap!

Of course, with all these opportunities, you might find that you start to take too much on. You want to help others, give your gifts to the world, and be a super-hero! You've sprouted and are finally blooming, but it still takes some time for petals to fully open. Be patient and mindful of overcommitting, since taking on too much is easy for many of us to do.

SUMMARY

Linear living neglects inner spring. Many people will jump into projects without intentional planning, then end up spinning in circles around distractions and unintended outcomes.

The beauty of cyclical living is that winter sets the scene, and spring strategizes what'll come next. Being intentional with each season's powers fuels impactful cycles, and the ideas and focus that spring brings will bring your big ideas to life.

If you find inner spring a fun season for you, consider how you can set up systems and processes into your life and work that enhance your talents. They don't have to look linear!

If inner spring is challenging for you, consider why. Is it a fear of visibility? Do you find anxiety in all the action? Consider what spring-influenced self-care tips can ground you during a sprouting season, and commit to making time for one each day.

● ● ●

MY SPRING ALMANAC

Use this worksheet to get to know *your* inner spring. Make a few copies to revisit the exercise over a few cycles.

1. Imagine Earth's season of spring. What words come to mind when you think about the energy behind springtime?

---

2. Considering the words you wrote down, what are some tiny ways you could enhance that energy in your everyday life?

---

3. What Cycle Days do you notice that you're in your inner spring? (Remember, Cycle Day 1 is the first day of your full flow period.)

---

4. Next time you find yourself in inner spring, note any obstacles that show up here:

---

5. And, jot down any personal strengths you notice come out:

---

6. While you're in your inner spring, brain dump all the things that sound appealing and fulfilling in this part of your cycle:

Review this worksheet each Spring for a few cycles to deeply understand what the season looks like for *you*.

●　　●　　●

CHAPTER 4

INNER SUMMER

● ● ●

Think about summer energy for a moment. How would you describe it?

The height of summer brings warmth, excitement, and abundance. Gardens burst with life, the days are long, and a sense of adventure and ease fill the air. The planet is at peak vitality and growth, shrouded in color. Maybe you feel the same way?

Cheers to inner summer! This is your ovulatory phase, or the time around ovulation, the release of an egg in your ovary. Many menstruators notice this season begins one to two weeks after the start of their period.

THE OVULATORY PHASE

Inner spring turns into inner summer as you approach ovulation. Your body is gearing up to release an egg in a few days, which is biologically the main event of your entire menstrual cycle.

From an evolutionary perspective, your estrogen peaks due to your mammalian brain's attempt to get you out in the world and flirting with potential mates, and peaking testosterone makes you competitive. Your follicles are growing, and one's about to release an egg, so you're at your most fertile. Consider what you're bringing to life—it doesn't have to be a baby! It could be a piece of art, a business, a relationship, even a book.

HOW YOU KNOW YOU'RE ENTERING INNER SUMMER

❁ There's a general excitement about your life!

❁ You feel able to communicate clearly and with ease.

❁ You feel unstoppable, energetic, flirty, and magnetic.

❁ You want to RSVP yes to all invitations.

❀ Your cervical mucus changes to slippery, stretchy, clear, or wet.

YOUR FULLEST OUTWARD EXPRESSION: DARE TO DREAM

Inner summer feels like you're in full bloom! You might feel a natural high, like anything is possible. It's like you're an elevated version of yourself. You might find that it's easy to take care of others, and you can serve others before having to take care of yourself (which likely wouldn't happen during inner winter). Even your body can handle more stress at this time in your cycle. You still want to get enough sleep (always!), but you can wake up earlier and likely still have good energy throughout the day. You're more resilient—take advantage of it!

Inner summer is the time to go after your goals. It's the time for broad, bold moves with which you can share your gifts with the world, especially since you can save any details or finesse for inner autumn. You'll be friendly and chatty, seeking connection with other people and collaboration on projects. Your inner critic is quieter, so you feel a sense of mastery and competence. This is the time to run the race, ask for a raise, go on a date, redecorate the home, and work on "the meat" of a project.

THE PRODUCTIVITY TRAP

When we believe that *doing more* will lead to more fulfillment, we gobble up more work. You pick up others' slack. You say yes to duties that don't deeply resonate with you. You may even get a reputation for being "the one who gets it done," the person who will always say yes. And it's all in the name of showing how productive and what a hard worker you are.

During inner summer, with all your confidence and ease, thoughts may creep into your mind, like, "Wow, I should always do this much each day!" or "Clearly I can handle more responsibilities; I just need to be more disciplined." In our culture, this hyper-hustle of summer energy is applauded.

The catch? This doesn't lead to fulfillment, after all. It leads to burnout and overwhelm. You've probably been there.

Next thing you know, you're sacrificing quality for quantity. You're skipping self-care. You ignore the creative side projects that truly excite you.

Yeah, summer can feel pretty dang awesome. But here's the thing—it's only a great phase because it's temporary. There's no endless summer; the seasons always change.

If you force yourself to stay constantly in a summer state, you will burn out. Nobody can be 100 percent on 100 percent of the time. The body, mind, and soul require periods of rest. Periods of lower productivity are what make the periods of higher productivity possible, just like with every cycle in nature.

Linear living expects you to perform as if it's summer all the time. But the secret of cyclical living is that you can get more done with less burnout, and less fighting your own body, since you work with the strengths of *each* season, not just summer's.

It's a good thing that inner summer doesn't last forever. Without the clarity and vision coming out of inner winter and the action plan designed in inner spring, you'd end up having nowhere to aim your energy. You need the rest of the seasons in order to best share your gifts with the world during inner summer. Each season has its purpose. Enjoy each of them.

THE MIDSUMMER SHIFT

You know how on the summer solstice, someone always has to come out of the woodwork to remind you that the days are getting shorter from that point on? (Thanks, dude.) Just as the other seasons, summer morphs over time. The dead of summer may be as hot and exciting as a fourth of July party, but at some point there's a subtle shift. Yes, the days are technically getting shorter. The early wildflowers lost their color. The initial rush of energy wanes a bit, but it's still high and stable.

The middle of your inner summer may be when the hormone progesterone enters the scene, shifting the feel of inner summer a bit. Remember, before ovulation, estrogen is your key hormone player. After ovulation (which for most menstruators is the peak of inner summer), progesterone becomes the dominant sex hormone, and you might feel the shift.

Progesterone—when your hormones are healthy—can help you feel calm, happy, and well. But it's a bit less buzzy than when your estrogen peaked shortly before. For example, I find that after ovulating, I'm still a social butterfly, prolific at work and excited about life for a few days, but it's through a more grounded, softer lens. Some menstruators have a different experience with this shift after ovulation, possibly feeling anxious or tired from it. Be aware that a shift happens, and see how it manifests in *your* body.

POWERS OF INNER SUMMER

CREATIVITY

Humans are creative by nature. And to take it further, nature *wants* you to be creative right now. Inner summer is the phase when conception is most likely to occur, after all. Thanks to the effects of estrogen and testosterone peaking at this time, you might feel peak motivation, inspiration, sensuality, and connection to your body, all excellent ingredients for creative work.

So whatever you feel called to create, make it, build it, do it! The world needs your creative talent. How can you add even 1 percent more of it to the world this cycle?

CHARM AND ATTRACTION

Again, your biology is trying to get you out and about in the world. Basically, nature wants to up your chances of finding a mate and reproducing. Not only is there fascinating research about your *appearance* changing when you're fertile (like facial symmetry, glowing skin, and full lips—but that's for another book), but also the feel-good hormone levels put an extra pep in your step.[3]

You carry yourself and walk with more confidence, which makes the rest of the world attracted to you (not just in a finding-a-mate way, in friendly and platonic ways, too!). The heightened confidence and socialness elevate your natural charm. Let them adore you!

PLEASURE

This high-hormone season allows you to feel good—really good. Not only might you notice pleasure from enhanced senses (like you're more sensitive to scents and notice tactile sensations more), but it's also when you're likely to feel most pleasure from sexual experiences.

Inner summer may be when you desire sex the most or find that it's the "best" at this time. In fact, some people feel a strong desire *only* around this time,

---

3 Roberts et al. "Female Facial Attractiveness Increases during the Fertile Phase of the Menstrual Cycle," *Proceedings of the Royal Society B-Biological Sciences* 271, Suppl 5 (August 7, 2004): S270-2, https://doi .org/10.1098/rsbl.2004.0174.

and that's okay! Find moments of pleasure, both big and small, throughout the whole season.

MASTERY

Inner summer can feel like reaping rewards without a ton of effort. You feel like you can do it all, and do it all well. Your work, communication, and relationships feel smoother. Your high self-esteem, energy, and confidence give you an air of ease, like you know you're great at what you do.

This season is excellent for getting in the zone with whatever you're up to, whether it's working, exercising, or running an event. Build in time for deep work to harness your mastery!

COMMUNICATION AND CONNECTION

Isn't it nice when words come super easily to you? You may notice that capability in inner summer. You speak with ease and your writing is more prolific. You feel like it's safe to put yourself out there, on a literal or metaphorical stage, to share ideas and link up with old and new connections.

This is the optimal time to show up on video, do public speaking, ask someone on a date, pitch work, network, ask for a big favor... the possibilities are endless. Find a way to get yourself in front of others and see what happens.

CHALLENGES OF INNER SUMMER

UNWANTED ATTENTION

Being so "seen" can be scary. Your powers in this season can make you extra visible. You might not want to share everything—to share *yourself*—with the world, but the world is more likely to notice you in your inner summer. Plus, if you're working through trauma or shame around something in your life, the extra attention can make you quite uncomfortable.

If you feel happier in the shadows of inner autumn and winter, inner summer might make you want to curl up and hide from it all. It's absolutely okay to schedule in plenty of alone time or to avoid busy social situations if you're not up for them. Prepare for these feelings in your schedule; take *yourself* on a date, set early bedtimes to restore yourself, have a close friend you can call whenever you're overwhelmed, and spend time in nature to feel the connection with the earth without being front and center in society.

LOST OPPORTUNITIES

You may want to do it all, but you obviously can't. For everything you say yes to, there's another opportunity you have to say no to. After all, life is a series of tradeoffs! This can bug the crap out of people in inner summer, when you tend to feel like anything is possible.

On the other side, you might groan at yourself if you don't let anything come to fruition during inner summer. Say you didn't set an intention in inner winter, or you didn't set a plan in inner spring. What exactly are you supposed to be working on with a purpose? Inner summering without intention might lead to feeling scattered, frustrated, or anxious since there's no meat of a project to work with. See? You truly do need every other season to enjoy inner summer.

SELF-CARE AND RITUALS TO TRY THIS CYCLE

Want to harness the excitement and adventure of summertime? You can build habits and rituals into this phase to stay grounded while going after your goals and intentions!

You might have a packed schedule this season, but you *can* prioritize time to care for yourself. Check out these ideas and consider what will keep up your excitement and gratitude while ensuring you don't burn out. Which one to three ideas could you try next inner summer?

HOW YOU CAN BEGIN TO EMBRACE INNER SUMMER

❀ Keep a gratitude list. Each morning, jot down something that you're grateful for, no matter how simple or grand it is.

❀ Keep a wins list! At the end of each day, write down a win from the day that highlights a great quality about yourself.

❀ Enjoy creative time, such as writing, crafts, or dancing. Find a way to express yourself through the process of creation!

❀ Find time—even just a few hours!—to spend with a loved one. For example, spend quality time with your partner—without the kids.

❀ Host a dinner party. Make it collaborative, like a potluck or a night of yard games.

❀ Organize your closet.

❀ Bring fresh flowers into the house.

- Find a private place to go skinny-dipping or sunbathing.
- Give yourself a massage with coconut oil and essential oils.
- Send a card to someone you love.
- Post the bold social media post you've been thinking about.
- Batch cook some meals to freeze for your late inner autumn.
- Take some fresh photos of yourself.
- Wear the bold dress or lipstick.
- Offer to host a party or get-together for a club or organization you belong to.
- Attend a charity event.

JOURNAL PROMPTS FOR INNER SUMMER

With all the meetings on your schedule, you might think you don't have time to sit down and write or reflect. Perhaps that's a sign you've overcommitted? Find time to ground yourself to ensure you're meeting your cycle's intention!

- Write a love letter to yourself to read later in your cycle.
- Who in your life is currently lighting up your soul?
- Describe a moment of pride or celebration that you've recently experienced.
- Do you have any big dreams or smaller goals that are coming together?
- Are you focusing too much energy on something that's not worth it?
- Check in with your intuition. Is there any wisdom you need to hear?
- How are you making the world a better place?

TRY IT: A TINY TWEAK FOR THE BUSY MENSTRUATOR

If you find that during inner summer, you sometimes forget to eat or rest during all the hustle and bustle, set daily reminders on your phone to remind you to take care of yourself.

THE CYCLE SYNCING HANDBOOK

TRY IT: A BOLD MOVE FOR THE
DEVOTED CYCLE SYNCER

Every cycle, find a time to spotlight one of your creations. It could be as simple as showing off a portfolio piece on LinkedIn or sending an email newsletter. Or, to go bigger, you might plan a workshop at the local library around one of your skills or pitch yourself as a guest on a podcast you love.

SUMMER'S LIFE LESSON:
LOG YOUR WINS

With so many bold moves happening in inner summer, you might easily let some of them slip away from your memory.

I noticed that whenever I needed evidence that I'm great at what I do, it was challenging to think of a specific example. Whether it's for a website testimonial or just a boost in daily happiness, keeping track of personal wins and positive feedback from others is now quick and super impactful.

I have a folder on my computer titled "Folder o' Wins." If someone sends me a kind message about myself or my work, I take a screenshot and upload it. If somebody emails me amazing feedback about a program or event I ran, I enter it on a spreadsheet organized by project. I even have a document called "Things People Say about Me" so that when I need to write a bio, I can pull from what others think!

Keeping a log of all your wins can change how you see yourself. And inner summer is a crucial time to track them. Take a few minutes every cycle to enter your wins from the past month. You'll be especially grateful in your inner autumn when you may need a confidence boost.

TAKE IT FURTHER: FIND
YOUR SPECIAL SAUCE

So often, we focus on the things we struggle with. We want to improve our weaknesses. Of course, this can be helpful at times. But what if we spent more time elevating what we're already great at instead?

When we work on what comes naturally to us, we're more likely to feel in flow and fully engaged. We might not even realize how skilled we are at an activity, since it feels effortless and fun! Ever think, "This can't be that good; I barely tried!" or "It doesn't count, it was too easy"? But those skills that feel easy to you aren't natural to everyone—they're *your* gifts. And by practicing them, you'll keep getting better.

So how can you stand out when you know what you're talented at? Think about this for a couple minutes: What are the things that you're better at doing compared to most people? You can certainly identify a few; everybody has at least a few areas where they'd land in the top third of a group.

Now, can you discover a *combination* of two things you're really great at? The more unique the combo, the better—because how many people on the planet could have the same mix? Maybe you're an excellent writer, but you're also an exceptional dancer. How many people can you name that are high-level writer-dancers? Maybe you're a great civil engineer at work, but you love story-telling and live performance. Could you be one of the top professional speakers at engineering conferences? Maybe you work as a yoga teacher but do photography on the side. Can you imagine how many yoga studios and retreat spaces could use your gifts? Are you a nurse who's a talented watercolor painter? Plenty of people could use some beautiful anatomy paintings.

When you discover your secret sauce, not only will you stand out from the crowd, but you'll also automatically be at the top of your field. Because you designed your own field.

Work hard on the things that come easy to you.

WHAT FELLOW MENSTRUATORS SAY

- ❀ "Ovulation is empowering. I feel more confident in this phase. To the extent that I ever get the 'I'm crushing life' feeling, it happens in this phase." —Dani
- ❀ "I feel refreshed and prepared to take on life's problems. I feel on top of the world and physically at my best." —Caitlin
- ❀ "My sense of smell is absurdly and annoyingly keen." —Amy

TRANSITIONING TO INNER AUTUMN

You may feel a transition away from inner summer's energy a few days after ovulation. It can be subtle, just like the days getting shorter after the summer solstice and the air cooling a bit toward the end of the planet's summer season.

It might continue to feel like inner summer for some days after ovulation, but the boldness might fade. Your cervical fluid dries up and thickens after ovulation, and you feel drier. You want more sleep and notice an increase in food cravings, or feel like you need more food, period.

For many, it might feel like a much-needed grounding, with anxiety or just too much stimulation finally easing off. Plenty of menstruators welcome this seasonal change once the transition passes.

SUMMARY

Many menstruators adore the inner summer season, since it feels most fruitful. After all, that's when we find fresh local fruit at the store and enjoy lush home gardens!

But remember: summer isn't endless, and nothing on Earth can bloom through all four seasons. The harvest will come, as will winter. Fully using inner spring's powers sets you up to do amazing work in inner summer, and you can harvest the results come inner autumn.

If inner summer is a fantastic time for you, think about how you can give more of your gifts to the world. Do you want to start a side project or business to share those strengths? Could you schedule cyclical volunteer work for this time?

If you struggle with elements of inner winter, reflect on which part is difficult to embrace. Do you feel like you have nothing to create? Maybe use your next inner winter to reflect on what you could bring to life in inner summer. Is all the attention uncomfortable for you? Find ways to be a powerful behind-the-scenes leader.

●　　●　　●

MY SUMMER ALMANAC

Use this worksheet to get to know *your* inner summer. Print a few copies to track your answers over a few months.

1. Imagine Earth's season of summer. What words come to mind when you think about the energy behind summertime?

---

2. Considering the words you wrote down, what are some tiny ways you could enhance that energy in your everyday life?

---

3. What Cycle Days do you notice that you're in your inner summer? (Remember, Cycle Day 1 is the first day of your full-flow period.)

---

4. Next time you find yourself in inner summer, note any obstacles that show up here:

---

5. Jot down any personal strengths you notice that come out during inner summer:

---

6. While you're in your inner summer, brain dump all the things that sound appealing and fulfilling in this part of your cycle:

Come back to this worksheet each inner summer for a few cycles, and you'll start to paint a very clear picture of what the season looks like for *you*.

● ● ●

CHAPTER 5

INNER AUTUMN

• • •

How would you describe the energy driving autumn?

When autumn approaches, the world starts to slow down again. Leaves turn golden and red, then gently fall to the ground, reminding us that change is the only constant. There's a crispness to the air, and animals start preparing for a colder season.

When you're in your inner autumn, it's also your premenstrual phase, or roughly the time after ovulation and until your next period.

THE LUTEAL PHASE

As inner summer ends and inner autumn begins, you move away from ovulation and return to an infertile phase. Biologically, your body is preparing for pregnancy, whether or not pregnancy is even possible in that particular cycle. So, your body slows down and asks you to tune back into yourself, rather than focusing on the outer world. You produce the hormone progesterone and your estrogen levels fall.

You may have heard of the nesting phase before a pregnant person goes into labor. They start tidying up the house, finishing projects, and generally preparing home for the addition of a baby. Even if conception didn't occur this cycle, you might feel the cyclical urge to nest at this time as your body approaches the end (and, of course, start) of another cycle.

HOW YOU KNOW YOU'RE ENTERING INNER AUTUMN

❀ You start to feel less in flow and your energy wanes from peak.

❀ You start to withdraw and seek more alone time.

- You feel more sensitive, both about what others say or think and toward your own self-talk.
- You feel less concerned about doing things for others and more preoccupied with focusing on yourself.
- Sexual desire and vaginal lubrication decrease.

THE MISUNDERSTOOD SEASON

Inner autumn gets a bad rap since it overlaps with the premenstrual time. In reality, it can be a lovely season for many menstruators—*if* your needs during this time are honored. Some people feel very much at home in their inner autumn, since progesterone has a calming nature (especially contrasted with the energy of peak estrogen, which can be anxiety-inducing to some).

But let's be real, society doesn't push a calm vibe, most of the time. Your body might want one thing, but the pressures of living in this world can lead you to mismanage yourself in this season. You wonder why you're feeling weaker in your workouts, why you're having cravings, and why you're irritable, yet you tend to push through it all, even if you suffer from it.

It's especially difficult if you were too scattered during inner summer and didn't produce anything for you to finish up in your inner autumn, leaving you feeling unproductive and inefficient. Remember, by using your powers correctly in the earlier seasons, you'll get the sense of accomplishment that you deserve (and crave) during inner autumn.

To add insult to injury, we're told to cover up and hide our negative feelings, and it doesn't help when people joke, "Are you PMSing?" when you simply express justified anger or annoyance (regardless of where you are in your cycle). To this day, the premenstrual week's reputation is less than glowing. But as more menstruators discover the powers of this season, we're changing the way the world sees this phase.

This season is all about truth, insight, and pruning your life like your garden. Your inner autumn directly asks you, "But what do you *really* think and feel?" The needs and feelings that you suppressed in the other seasons come back to the surface, and the tasks you neglected arise. You can no longer ignore the tough parts of life, but that's a good thing—it's a chance to meet them head-on, come to resolutions, and grow. When you learn to use the strengths of inner autumn, you'll feel more powerful and grounded, which will make your contributions to yourself and the world more impactful.

PRUNE YOUR LIFE

When you prune a garden, you let the most important plants grow and bloom. Think about it: You prune weeds that you don't want hanging around, making space for the colorful blooms you love. That's how it works in your life, too. If you can prune in your inner autumn, then what really matters to you will bloom strong and healthy in future seasons.

Winter was about planting the seeds, spring letting them sprout, summer letting them bloom, and autumn allowing you to choose what to keep and what's in the way. The thorns that were obscured by roses are now visible, and you need to figure out what to do with them.

So, in the spirit of pruning, use inner autumn to determine new boundaries, clean up what you've outgrown, and look at things rationally, which, let's be honest, you couldn't do as well in inner summer. In fact, inner autumn's the best decision-making phase of your cycle, since your instincts are sharper, you're more intuitive, and you're less impulsive. You can deeply analyze all options and come to a confident decision. Plus, you'll naturally crave order, completion, and clarity, which is a great plus when wrapping up work projects or tackling household tasks. What a fantastic opportunity not only to decide what matters most, but also to get it *done*.

So, prune away!

THAT INNER CRITIC IN YOUR HEAD

There it is... that voice in your head that pops up every once in a while to tell you what a bad job you're doing. "Who are you to think you could accept that board position?" "You should've been able to make that catch, just get off the field." "Ew, what are you wearing?" "They did that way better than you." "Why did you say that? You're so embarrassing."

Ouch. We all hear it from time to time, but your inner critic tends to come most alive during inner autumn. You can certainly tell it to pipe down when needed, but here's the fascinating secret of your inner critic: although what it says may sound sharp and rude, if you pull back some layers, you may find a kernel of insight that's truly helpful to think about.

Sure, its voice might sound dramatic, but could there perhaps be a teeny bit of truth to what it's saying? Can you dig out the core of what your critic is trying to tell you, and throw away the rest? What is the single grain of truth amid the sassy attitude? This is your time to get deep. Get dark, if you feel like it. Dig, dig,

dig to figure out what the nugget of wisdom is that that voice is trying to tell you, even though it's doing it rudely.

Often, your inner critic is just trying to protect you from past hurts. It wants to take care of you by helping you find truth and improvement. It's a sign that you're growing out of your comfort zone (which is a good thing). It's just one part of your whole self.

Remember, whatever you're feeling is information. Information leads to knowledge, and knowledge leads to empowerment. Get used to questioning yourself and finding the root of your thoughts, along with a healthy dose of self-compassion. Inner autumn builds emotional intelligence, if you let it. Uncover the dirt and find the diamonds.

POWERS OF INNER AUTUMN

TRUTH SPEAKING

With heightened clarity and honesty at this time, you may find it easier to discover your needs and speak your truth. Remember, your inner critic gets louder during your autumn, and so does your intuition. Find out what they want. It's incredibly empowering, since you can set boundaries, make decisions, and assert yourself in a way that feels authentic and aligned with your values. You can be fantastic at standing up for yourself here.

You also feel more confident with sharing criticism with others, since you see problems clearly without the rose-colored glasses of inner summer. Of course, share mindfully and constructively. Not everyone is in the straight-speaking, no-nonsense phase that you are in. Respond, don't react.

EDITING AND ORGANIZING

All that detail-oriented work that's been piling up? Now's the time! You spent time earlier this cycle understanding the big picture, and now you get the added benefit of paying attention to the details so you can finesse the project. Plus, the clarity of this season helps you prioritize, make decisions, and stay on track.

Put that strategic thinking to good use when it comes to deep focus work in the first half of your autumn. In the second half, as your energy wanes, use your organizing powers to do tasks that take less brainpower, like cleaning your kitchen or going through your inbox—necessary to-dos that seem more appealing in this season.

REFOCUSING AND COMPLETION

In inner autumn, you'll have an itch to wrap everything up and bring projects to a close. But before you prune and tend, take a step back to assess the full situation. Gain perspective around what needs to be focused on first, and what can wait. Reflect on what's happened in the past weeks, evaluate progress toward goals, and figure out what needs adjusting. Get rid of what's not working, and take inventory of what is.

Then, get to work! Keep the distractions at bay and you can be super productive in this season, using your focus, deep thought, and purposeful work to bring projects to completion. Your body is preparing for the end of a cycle, so you have an inborn urgency to finish up. It's like an internal deadline motivating you to keep going.

INNER GUIDANCE AND DISCERNMENT

Often, you'll finally feel like a true grown-up in this phase, mature and able to get real. You can rationally look at a situation with fresh eyes, without the giddiness of inner summer obscuring it. After letting an idea mull around for most of a cycle, you may finally get more clarity around a decision you've been sitting on (or, maybe your gut tells you you need to wait another cycle).

You can more easily decide what's for you, and what's not. When your inner guidance tells you to say no, that's a good thing. After doing so much for others, your body is reminding you to focus on the goals you set for yourself. Remember, a no in one place means a yes somewhere else.

WILDNESS

One of the most overlooked powers of the entire cycle is your ability to connect with your wild self. You can feed the primitive, raw, and free spirit deep inside you, as if you're living in the wild at one with nature and yourself.

You've likely been conditioned by society to be prim, proper, and perfect—screw all that! A little chaos is beautiful; destruction is a natural part of many natural cycles. This is your cyclical reminder to make a mess, live like a river undammed, and connect with what it really feels like to be a cycling human; every cycle gives you more life experience, making you wiser and more wild.

CHALLENGES OF INNER AUTUMN

LOW SELF-ESTEEM

Beyond the inner critic, you may struggle with other premenstrual mood-related symptoms. Your body image hits a low, you're overly self-conscious, you nitpick at yourself, and you might experience anxiety, depression, or overwhelm. You could struggle with impostor syndrome or social media comparison.

As much as possible during inner autumn, avoid anything that depresses you. Scrolling on your phone? Watching the news? Listening to a friend complain? You can certainly take a break for a few days and find something that lights you up to fill the time. Plus, before doing big things in your inner autumn—like a presentation, performance, or meeting—you might need more of a pep talk than usual. You're also more likely to have vulnerability hangovers!

PHYSICAL WOES

Most menstruators experience at least one premenstrual symptom, but premenstrual physical tension, discomfort, and pain exist on a spectrum. Intensity varies based on your genetics, stress, nutrient deficiencies, thyroid health, gut health, and hormone levels, among other factors. Please note that *normal* symptoms should be mild enough that you can still live your life; you don't have to change plans or stay home for days. Pain or discomfort that affects your life significantly isn't normal and should be brought to the doctor.

Common PMS complaints include cramping, bloating, pain in the lower back, appetite changes, stomach upset, acne, headaches or migraines, sleep issues, anxiety, sore breasts, fatigue, low libido, mood changes (anger, irritability), brain fog, and just feeling the blues. If any of these significantly interfere with your life, it'll be hard to embrace this part of your cycle at *all*—and it definitely warrants medical care.

A SHARP TONGUE

The flip side of your truth-telling power is coming off as rude or hostile. You might let raw thoughts and feelings slip out without being mindful, which can come off as *brutally* honest or disrespectful. Why do we often assume that others know what we're thinking? Why do we get mad that they can't read our minds? Instead, we can use our powers to carefully craft how we communicate in inner autumn.

Of course, we all get impatient and frustrated from time to time. Keep it at a minimum by staying on top of your inner autumn self-care: avoid getting hangry, get enough sleep, and take regular breaks. Don't let those pent-up feelings explode.

SELF-CARE AND RITUALS TO TRY THIS CYCLE

The inward draw of autumn can certainly make you crave intentional moments of self-care. You've done a lot of work over the past couple weeks, and it's time to pull back a bit so you can prepare for a much-deserved rest.

Review the self-care tips below; what would make sense in your life? Decide on one to three action points to start implementing next inner autumn.

HOW YOU CAN BEGIN TO EMBRACE INNER AUTUMN

- ❁ Satisfy your needs before those of others.
- ❁ Simplify your schedule. Nix any plans that aren't essential or exciting.
- ❁ Deep-clean your home. Recycle or give away any junk building up.
- ❁ Add in extra sleep, especially if you need to catch up. Schedule naps into your day, if you're a nap person.
- ❁ Set your work hours for when you feel best. You might find that a later work schedule is better in this season.
- ❁ Brain dump all your wishes, fears, concerns, and ideas. Let it all out when you're feeling overwhelmed! Then, stash the paper until your next inner spring so you can use fresh eyes to determine what needs to be addressed and what can be scrapped.
- ❁ Write down a reminder on your calendar or put a sticky note on your laptop that says, "It's okay to say no," or any other reminder you need.
- ❁ Add new boundaries wherever needed.
- ❁ Catch up on a book you're in the middle of.
- ❁ Sort through photos and delete what you don't need.
- ❁ Get some endorphins from a good workout. Try a long bike ride or paddle.
- ❁ Spend intimate time with a partner, and move slowly.
- ❁ Ask for what you want, clearly and confidently.
- ❁ Create a feel-good space in your home.

- Take note of your transition days from inner summer to inner autumn and from inner autumn to inner winter so they don't catch you off guard and leave you feeling self-critical.
- Take a true lunch break, away from your desk and technology, ideally outdoors.
- Use a sunrise-imitating alarm clock, or get outside as soon as possible after waking.
- Have a solo dance party to work out any anger or frustration.
- Take an Epsom salt bath.

JOURNAL PROMPTS FOR INNER AUTUMN

As you turn inward and bring deep truths and insights to mind, take time to record and reflect so you can truly apply your wisdom.

- What is a decision you've been procrastinating on? Can you find some clarity?
- Is there anything that isn't lighting up your life like you expected it to?
- Describe any fears or limiting beliefs you've been holding. Can you let them go?
- Have you been doing anything that doesn't feel authentically you?
- Are you focusing too much on something that makes you angry or frustrated?
- What needs do you have this week, and what boundaries do you need to draw?
- How can you best support yourself between now and your period?

. . . .

TRY IT: A TINY TWEAK FOR THE BUSY MENSTRUATOR

During your inner autumn, go to bed 20 minutes earlier than usual. That's it. Promise you'll do it? Cool.

. . . .

TRY IT: A BOLD MOVE FOR THE
DEVOTED CYCLE SYNCER

Ready to prune your to-do list and use your discernment power?
Try the ABCDE Method. List out all the to-dos still on your plate
at this point in your cycle. Then, assign a letter to each. A tasks
are important and time-sensitive; you need to get to them by
the end of the cycle at the latest. B tasks are important but
less time-sensitive; you can get around to them next cycle, if
need be. C tasks are the nice-to-haves, D tasks can be given to
someone else (did you over-commit again?), and E tasks can
simply be crossed out. They're clearly not urgent or important!

INNER AUTUMN'S LIFE LESSON:
THE POWER OF HELP

One of the most vulnerable things we can do as humans is to ask for help. Especially in today's society, we're expected to be self-sufficient, to pull ourselves
up by our own bootstraps and figure it out ourselves so we don't appear weak.

But in the last few days of the cycle, late in inner autumn, your energy wanes.
You might have a lot left on your plate, especially if your work or family don't
allow for much in the way of cyclical living. Maybe you deal with physical or
mental premenstrual symptoms, and when an inconvenience needs addressing, you *literally can't even.*

Of all the seasons, inner autumn is the one in which you're most likely to act
when you feel that urge to reach out to someone—a friend, partner, parent, or
even a stranger—for help. Inner autumn is also when you get crystal clear on
what you need and how you need it—which makes it an excellent time to practice asking for support.

You might not feel like you need to ask for help as much in inner spring or
inner summer. I'd bet you *give* help a lot in those weeks, though. And there are
countless menstruators in their spring or summer while you're in your autumn
and winter, ready and excited to give you their help. Use it—it helps you while
making them feel good, too!

THE CYCLE SYNCING HANDBOOK

The perks of getting great at asking for support? You open your eyes to new perspectives and knowledge. You might find a new solution you hadn't considered. You build deeper relationships and connections with others. You empower yourself and others to take action and seek resources. And, of course, you can release some stress and anxiety, which will make inner autumn way more fun!

When you need (or just want) to ask for help, be, choose the right person to ask (based on their skill, availability, and willingness), express your gratitude, and give yourself compassion. Remember, help is a two-way street. You can return the favor to your helper later.

TAKE IT FURTHER: CELEBRATING YOUR WINS

As a society, we struggle with celebrating ourselves or even simply being proud of our own accomplishments. It's easy to cheer on a friend when they finish a race, get a promotion, or bring a creative project to life, but when it's ourselves? Not so easy.

But if your self-confidence takes a dip in your inner autumn, reminding yourself of accomplishments from past seasons can give you a little (or big) boost.

As someone who loves the journey toward audacious goals in the outdoors and in work, I sometimes struggle with feeling unsatisfied after a big accomplishment. I might smile for just a moment before thinking, "Cool, what's next?" and moving onto planning my next adventure.

But what should I do? Throw a party? Brag on Instagram? It can feel awkward to celebrate yourself! What I've found works for me is purchasing a small memento of sorts that I truly adore, then dedicating that item to the memory of my accomplishment.

For example, after my first 50k run, I bought a pair of earrings. They're simple, mini, sparkly hoops that were less than $30. When I hit "Add to Cart," I intentionally thought of them as "my 50k earrings." Now, every time I wear them, I think about the accomplishment of finishing my first 50k.

Celebration is a part of the cycle of accomplishment. You set your goal, you strategize toward it, you achieve it, and then you celebrate and reflect. Skipping celebration is like skipping the inner autumn of goal setting. Try it out: next time you make something BIG happen, can you find a little item to remind you to be proud of it? (But also, a party and Instagram brag totally work as well.)

WHAT FELLOW MENSTRUATORS SAY

❀ "I feel two strong but opposing urges—the first one is to clean and purge my space, followed shortly by the urge to draw inward and rest. I'm my most accepting of my body's boundaries and limitations during this phase." —Amy

❀ "I think of this phase as a time to slow down and complete anything unfinished." —Rachel

❀ "I get acne and bloating around ovulation, so I love when that clears up in autumn." —Elle

TRANSITIONING BACK TO INNER WINTER

As always, your cycle experience is unique. Many menstruators find that inner winter comes with their period or starts a couple days before bleeding. You might feel changes in your body that mean your period is coming soon; that might mark your transition to inner winter. If you chart your cycles, you could see your basal body temperature decrease. Maybe you see spotting. Some people feel like they're bleeding even if they're not yet, or feel a heaviness in their abdomen. A sudden drop in bloating, breast tenderness, and other tension can signal an impending change.

Mentally, you might feel a sense of nearing an end of sorts, or a feeling of release. You might not feel like making any further progress on projects, like you did what you could and now it's time to step back.

The transition to inner winter can bring relief for many, but it may bring pain or discomfort for others who struggle with their periods. Use this transition time to prepare for what you know you'll need in your inner winter.

SUMMARY

Being mindful of cyclical living can ease the premenstrual phase for many menstruators. Inner autumn is a misunderstood season, since it's a phase of slowing down, which society doesn't typically encourage. Remember, linear living often revolves around trying to force yourself into an eternal summer (leading to burnout, naturally).

The truth is that by honoring a cyclical lifestyle—making space for times of push *and* pull, high *and* low—you'll welcome the effects of inner autumn, since you realize it's necessary to uncover the strengths of the other three seasons.

If you find inner autumn to be a lovely season, can you identify boundaries that you can honor at other times of your cycle?

If inner autumn is a rough time for you, determine whether the challenges stem from physical or mental (or both) causes. Physical symptoms that surpass mild should be taken seriously by healthcare providers, so start collecting data now. Have decent physical experiences, but struggle with the self-critic? Review the autumn-inspired self-care strategies and experiment with what helps ease it.

●　　●　　●

MY INNER AUTUMN ALMANAC

Use this worksheet to get to know *your* inner autumn. Photocopy the exercise so you can track patterns over your next few cycles.

1. Imagine Earth's season of autumn. What words come to mind when you think about the energy behind fall?

----

2. Considering the words you wrote down, what are some tiny ways you could enhance that energy in your everyday life?

----

3. What Cycle Days do you notice that you're in your inner autumn? (Remember, Cycle Day 1 is the first day of your full-flow period.)

----

4. Next time you find yourself in inner autumn, note any obstacles that show up here:

_____

_____

_____

_____

5. Jot down any personal strengths that you notice come out in your inner autumn:

_____

_____

_____

_____

6. While you're in your inner autumn, brain dump all the things that sound appealing and fulfilling in this part of your cycle:

_____

_____

_____

_____

Come back to this worksheet each inner autumn for a few cycles, and you'll start to paint a very clear picture of what the season looks like for _you_.

●　●　●

CHAPTER 6

CREATIVITY, WORK, AND YOUR CYCLE

● ● ●

I used to think that all "productivity" meant was getting things done, checking items off a to-do list, and doing it all quickly. With that mindset, I felt like I was in a constant state of hustle, doing the absolute most I could (even if quality—or my brainpower—suffered).

I voluntarily accepted new projects, even if I was in the thick of others that I was more passionate about. I scheduled events for days when I already knew I'd feel like crap. Heck, at my most chaotic, I made to-do lists *of to-do lists* that I knew I had to write!

Like so many other humans living the grind, I burned out. I wondered where my passion and inspiration had gone, why I had no patience during meetings, and why I woke up dreading turning on the computer. It seemed like no matter what, I'd have to do tasks each day that would insidiously make me hate my job. I'd spend way too long searching for new jobs, even though I knew I wouldn't realistically leave my own at that time. I wondered whether I should go to grad school, or whether I should sell everything I owned and travel on pennies instead.

That period of my career happened to overlap with when I began to learn about my body's cyclical nature. As becoming more in tune with your body tends to teach you, I started to pick up on energy patterns and key moments of motivation. By noticing what came easily (and what came with more difficulty) to me at different times over the weeks and months, I had an *aha* moment: I didn't hate my work, but I needed to organize and schedule it more creatively.

Jumping into an experiment, I started making whatever work tasks I could cyclical. In my inner winter, I'd review the goals I'd set before, check my progress, and adapt objectives when necessary. When inner spring arrived, I'd start new projects, do research, and outline creative work. I got the bulk of my creative work (and networking) done in inner summer. Once inner autumn rolled around, I got to the mundane but focused-required tasks like expense reports, budgeting, and billing.

It's not like my work drastically changed; I still had to attend meetings I didn't want to and accept projects I didn't have time for. But I felt more joyful at work knowing that I had a reason for feeling the way I did, that I didn't have to do the same things in the same way every single day, and that I could plan my work wherever possible to better align with my energy and hormonal patterns. Even with managers and bureaucracy, these small alignments to my cycle helped me to feel less stressed and more inspired at work.

When I finally went full-time self-employed, I got the freedom to go even further with syncing my work to my cycle. That's when Ulysses Press reached out about writing this book. And you know what? I took an entire cycle to determine whether or not it was a project I wanted to pursue. In my inner spring, I outlined ideas and questions to ask the publisher. In my inner summer, I confided in a couple friends and a coach about the decision so I could talk it out. In my inner autumn, I created a pros and cons list and considered what I'd have to give up in order to write. By the time my inner winter rolled in, I had my answer: Yes, I wanted to write this book. And, in my heart, I knew the reasons why. It felt both intuitive and well-thought-out to wait for a complete cycle in order to make this choice.

What's been the most freeing is trusting the creative process. In fact, while writing this book, I took a month off of *everything* in my everyday life to go boating through the Grand Canyon. It was my longest chunk of consecutive time off the grid to date, and just six weeks before my manuscript was due.

Since I knew I'd be entirely disconnected from my usual life—like with no cell service, electricity, or contact with friends at home—I was curious to see if the experience of my cycle would be different from usual. Altogether, I started the trip in my luteal phase, got my period part way through, and finished the trip approaching ovulation.

But the interesting part to me was that the entire three weeks on the river felt like a lengthened inner winter. There was so much time simply to be present, intuitive, and without giant to-do lists. It was *not* a time to make plans, set goals, or analyze projects. It was extraordinarily refreshing, even though I knew I was quickly approaching the manuscript due date and still needed to, you know, write a casual *thirty-five thousand words*.

I was a bit concerned that I'd get home and have a hard time adjusting back to work life or wouldn't feel inspired after so long away. But it turns out, the inner summer and autumn I experienced after returning home were extremely fulfilling. Even though I dove hard back into my packed non-river life, I was able to seamlessly catch up on work, attend events, and make some exciting new connections throughout inner summer. Premenstrually, I had laser-sharp focus, solid discernment, and a calm demeanor at home. Those first weeks back were two of the most enhanced seasons I'd had in a very long while.

I shouldn't have been surprised! I'd let myself fully sink into an extended inner winter throughout the Grand Canyon, which is what allowed me to harness fully the potency of an inner summer and inner autumn dying to be expressed. Although I practice these concepts every cycle, it sometimes still catches me off guard to see how much the creative process *works*. By allowing regular rest and renewal, I opened up space for inspiration, motivation, clear creative analysis, and a massive dose of get-it-done-and-do-it-well attitude. Each season is vital to the harmony of the whole. And extended breaks can give you a big boost when you come out of creative hibernation.

And *that's* what productivity means to me now: allowing your body to share what it needs, and maximizing the energy it gives you. You might be like me, experiencing maximum productivity by embracing recurring bursts and rests.

LINEAR WORKFLOW	CYCLICAL WORKFLOW
Writing 1,000 words per day and sticking to a strict schedule, no matter your energy levels	Writing 5,000 words in a day when you get a burst of inspiration, and not writing at all when you don't feel creative
Moving that same item on your to-do list from one day to the next, until you get to it	Strategically scheduling and batching work for times you'll be most primed to do certain tasks
Jumping into work without allowing for research or planning	Allocating protected time for brainstorming, strategizing, communicating, and reflection around one project to improve over time

CREATIVE CYCLE MEETS MENSTRUAL CYCLE

Have you ever considered that the menstrual cycle is the ultimate act of creation? The menstrual cycle is designed to create new *life*! It's in our very nature to be creative.

But whether or not you want to have or currently have children, creativity isn't, of course, only about reproduction. You can use your cycle to create nearly anything: a project, a piece of art, a relationship, a community, a goal.

Everyone's creative; it's simply how you express who you are in the world! If you're thinking, "Nope, I'm just not a creative person!" I urge you to consider the fact that modern society (unrealistically) expects humans to be stuck in inner summer all the time, even though that's impossible. Big industry wants us to be in create mode 24/7, focusing on a product instead of the entire creative process that makes true innovation possible.

You can learn your creative ebbs and flow. It can be as simple as noting your energy highs and lows for certain tasks over the course of an entire cycle.

Then, you can apply what you know about your energy fluctuations to your work schedule.

In this cycle syncing framework, the seasons line up with the creative cycle like this:

CREATIVE CYCLE MEETS MENSTRUAL CYCLE

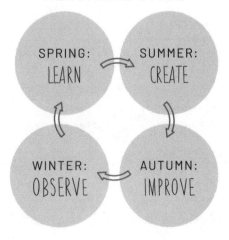

SPRING: LEARN

SUMMER: CREATE

WINTER: OBSERVE

AUTUMN: IMPROVE

THE CYCLE SYNCING HANDBOOK

The way your hormones ebb and flow across the four phases of your cycle affects your mental processes, motivation, and attitude. Doing what you can to cycle sync your work and projects can help you feel more inspired and focused. See what I mean about balancing your strengths? Each phase balances out the others and perfectly sets you up for the next.

Let's take a deeper look into the seasons and what you may be primed for, or struggling with, in each. As you read the following sections, you'll find tasks that you can lean into to enhance your inner season's powers, the tasks to avoid by scheduling them for a different time when you know you'll be happier doing them, and how to practice self-care at work. If your job has very limited flexibility or creativity, those self-care points might be your key to adding a bit of a cyclical nature to your otherwise linear work!

INNER WINTER: OBSERVE

In inner winter, your intuition will be strong and you will be able to think clearly about your desires and needs. In addition to reflecting deeply and collecting inspiration, pursuing quiet, solo, simple tasks can feel good at this time. So may taking an honest look at your current thoughts and feelings about your role and organization. You might even think of changes to suggest to your manager (or to commit to yourself) about your current projects or schedule.

You know when you have a gut feeling that something isn't quite right with a project? That'll surely bubble up to the surface during your menstrual phase. You don't have those pesky, high-energy hormones messing with your brain yet!

LEAN INTO
* Setting and reviewing goals (both short and long term)
* Taking a mental summary of all current projects to see what's aligning and what's not
* Evaluating whether your career is heading where you want it to
* Determining whether you need to ask for changes to your work situation (hours, location, duties, etc.)
* Simple, routine tasks (sending mail, reading newsletters in your inbox)

AVOID WHEN POSSIBLE

❀ Projects that require high energy or many people

❀ Meetings or presentations where you need to be ON for a large group

❀ Skipping lunch. (Take a real break to recharge!)

SELF-CARE PRACTICES

❀ If you have painful or uncomfortable periods, see if it's possible to work from home one to two days per cycle.

❀ Bring your favorite tea to your workspace when you need a pick-me-up.

❀ End your workday at its scheduled time. The rest can wait until your follicular phase.

INNER SPRING: LEARN

Get out the planner and sticky notes! During inner spring, you'll be able to approach what you're working on from new angles, and you might think of ideas you can't believe you hadn't thought of before. You'll become more extroverted and willing to try new things, so explore what's asking for your attention. You'll enjoy Happy Hour more at this time and will be excited to collaborate with other teams. It's the perfect time to plan out the next few weeks, since your brain wants to be intentional around the future.

LEAN INTO

❀ Planning out the rest of the cycle. Update your calendar, schedule meetings and projects, and get a networking event on the schedule for the next week.

❀ Any projects that are really exciting you

❀ Exploring new angles to approach a project or solve a problem

❀ Sharing what you're working on with others

AVOID WHEN POSSIBLE

❀ Letting impostor syndrome get to you. (Big idea? You can and already are doing it!)

❀ Overwhelming yourself with too many ideas. Keep a running list for when you have more time.

❀ Committing to too many plans for the rest of the cycle. Remember, in a couple weeks you won't want to attend *all* the things!

SELF-CARE PRACTICES

❀ Find a social opportunity. Organize a happy hour, find an event in your industry, or take a course for professional development.

❀ Keep nutritious snacks nearby. You might get so caught up in what you're doing that you'll forget to eat, or rely on snacks in the break room!

❀ Saying no if a task isn't a good fit. People will notice your increased energy and ask for a favor, but you won't have as much energy later this cycle—so plan accordingly.

INNER SUMMER: CREATE

Now's the time to really perform at work. Go the extra mile on projects you're loving, get the photo shoot, give your biggest presentations, and reach to exceed your goals. You'll be naturally more attractive to people, so go after what you want. Ask for the raise, meet with a VIP, suggest a bold pivot.

Do what you can to plan your most important presentations and meetings since both your communication skills and your charm will be highest here. It's also the time to be bold and ask for a raise or interview for a new position.

LEAN INTO

❀ Tackling the meat of projects. You did the planning in the follicular phase, so now it's time to execute it!

❀ Events and meetings involving lots of people

❀ Tasks that make you shine and call attention to your success

❀ Working on the hardest part of a project. (Your extra brainpower will give you a boost.)

AVOID WHEN POSSIBLE

❀ Burning out by not resting at all. You still need time to relax and recharge!

❀ Work that is slow-paced or not time-sensitive. You'll want ACTION.

❀ Getting TOO bold. Remember what your goals and dreams are (you thought of them during your menstrual phase) and focus on what will actually get you there.

SELF-CARE PRACTICES

❀ Taking short breaks to let out extra energy (like a quick walk or stretch)

❀ Having lunch with a colleague or someone in your industry

❀ Keeping your desk relatively organized. With so much going on, it's easy to let it get too messy!

INNER AUTUMN: IMPROVE

Ah, when your true feelings come out during a meeting. I've been there. Actually, I go there every month. This is when you really think critically about projects and start calling out issues as you see them. You'll head back toward more introversion and a no-nonsense mood during projects that frustrate you. But luteal phase thoughts are so valuable; you're able to point out flaws that somebody in the ovulatory phase wouldn't see.

So, use your inner autumn for revising, reorganizing, and wrapping up projects. You'll want to analyze, make decisions ,and think critically. You might feel most productive doing solo work; in inner autumn, you can get as much done as you did in inner summer, but it's more behind the scenes and could be less collaborative.

In fact, it's an excellent time for getting things *done*. Your brain wants you to wrap up as much as you can. So, revisit those unfinished projects and decide which are worth wrapping up, and which need a new direction (you can revisit them next cycle). Speaking of, you'll likely even feel an urge to tidy up and clean your workspace!

LEAN INTO

❀ Making crucial decisions

❀ Meeting deadlines

❀ Analytical tasks

❀ Reorganizing your notes, files, and desk

❀ Clearing out your inbox

AVOID WHEN POSSIBLE

❀ Starting brand-new projects. (You'll be more open to them in a couple weeks.)

❀ Tasks that involve a lot of creativity or teamwork

❀ Letting your emotions get the best of you (by snapping at others or feeling upset with your performance)

❀ Comparing yourself to your past work or to other people

SELF-CARE PRACTICES

❀ Setting visible boundaries when you don't want to be interrupted (like a color code, a sign, or a banner at your cubicle)

❀ Keeping items or decor in your workspace that make you happy or inspire you

❀ Taking mini solo breaks between meetings to mentally refresh by yourself

❀ Grabbing one of your favorite treats if you hit a rough day. Sometimes, a cappuccino and a scone can save the day.

CYCLICAL WORKFLOWS FOR PRODUCTIVITY

Whether or not you're able to align your work habits fully with your menstrual cycle, you can implement methods and tools to work more cyclically. Here are a few you can try.

TASK BATCHING

Batching your work can help you create a weekly or monthly workflow rather than having to give time every single day to a certain task. It involves collecting a set of tasks that are similar or related in some way, then executing them all in one set period.

Consider a social media manager. They *could* log on every single day to create a graphic or video on social media, think of a call to action, and write an applicable caption. Or, they could batch each part of the social media strategy. For example, they might spend one full day a month mapping out content ideas for the next month, one week filming content and collecting photos, a scheduled six-hour block for writing captions, and another scheduled day to proofread and schedule the content.

Or think of an accountant. They could allocate Mondays as their budget review day, Tuesdays as receipt processing day, and Wednesday as client meeting day. A writer might batch three to five blog posts at once and devote another period of time to editing them, rather than trying to write-edit, write-edit, write-edit. A software developer might schedule a different day to focus on a different feature of a new app. A teacher can set aside one day a week to grade papers all at once, instead of scattering them throughout the week. You might even notice this when you make appointments with others; ever notice how your doctor is only available certain days of the week?

Task batching decreases "task switching," or having to refocus whenever you shift your attention to a new task, which takes more time. Instead of constantly switching your brain's focus to a different task, you can fully sink into flow around one particular activity to minimize refocus time. The extra perk? When you can task batch according to your menstrual cycle, you can schedule batch work for when you feel most primed for certain tasks.

A+B WEEKS

If you can't or don't want set periods of task batching, you might decide to look on a bigger scale. Think about two different categories of your work, and when you can focus on each category. Alternating weeks can help you dedicate time to both the inward- and outward-facing duties of your work.

For example, your "A weeks" might be for anything collaborative and outward facing: client meetings, making sales, attending events, marketing, etc. Meanwhile, "B weeks" might be for deep, solo work time, plus administrative tasks, finances, reviewing progress, etc.

You can align this concept to your cycle by considering how you feel in each season. Perhaps you want your inner spring and autumn to be A weeks, and your inner summer and winter to be B weeks. You pick what works for you!

THEMED WEEKS

Similarly, instead of having two categories of weeks, you might assign a different theme for each week of a month. You could do this on a calendar, with each of the four full weeks of the month assigned around a particular type of work and the last few days for wiggle room. Or, you could design it around your menstrual cycle. For example, if you look at the month ahead, you might theme your inner summer week as your presentations and networking week.

You can theme your weeks on a month-to-month basis so you can adjust based on the current projects on the table. Or, depending on your work, you might even designate certain themes to certain weeks every single month. Maybe Week 2 is always about content creation, and Week 4 is for pitching and outreach every month. Play around and see what feels good to you.

SCHEDULE ADJUSTMENTS

Notice changes in energy throughout the day? Schedule for it! Perhaps in inner spring and summer, you feel like you can roll out of bed early and immediately dig into work, but in inner autumn and winter you get work done better in the afternoon and need your mornings for self-care. That's great data; plan ahead for it. Maybe one week per month, shift a workday to be a couple hours later than usual.

If your work requires you to be in an office or at a desk the exact same time every day, try to avoid scheduling meetings at inopportune times and batch work that'll feel better based on your energy fluctuations.

KNOWING THE WHY

As a part of the Observe phase of the creative process, or as part of your inner winter, can you get crystal clear on the Why behind your work?

When I start a new project (even when I began to write this book!), I like to write down the top three reasons why I want to finish the project, and do it well. Whenever my motivation fades, I scroll up to look at my Why, and it fuels me to keep going, even when it gets tedious.

What are the top three reasons you want to complete whatever you're working on? Put them in the header of your draft, write them on a sticky note at your desk, save them as your desktop background—whatever you need to do to reference them!

DO NOT DISTURB

Ever put your phone on DND? Many smartphones can set *multiple* DND settings. You can set different ones for different times. There are some days (and weeks) when I want email notifications to come through, and other times that I don't. Some days I work later than others, and so I adjust my notification settings to align with it.

Experiment with what settings you need in each phase. You might want to silence all notifications in your inner autumn, for example, when the last thing you want is to lose time mindlessly scrolling social media. Maybe you turn *on* certain notifications in your inner summer when you want more collaboration. The technology is there; play around.

VISUAL CUES FOR COWORKERS

When I worked in an office, I got fed up with the constant (though well-meaning) interruptions from colleagues. A manager suggested I craft a "traffic light" to show when I was available to chat. All I had to do was move a clothespin on some colored construction paper that I threw together; the "green light" meant I was available to chat or help. The "yellow light" meant that I could answer questions, but that I couldn't chat about non-work topics or get deep in conversation. The "red light" signaled to colleagues that they should only interrupt me in cases of emergency. They knew just by looking above my desk that they could come back later, at a time that worked for *both* of us.

I've met other people who have used a banner that they can clip across their cubicle to metaphorically "close the door," and others who have a sign that states that if their noise-canceling headphones are on, they are unavailable. You can work with your team or manager to determine a strategy that works for your workplace, and perhaps set a percentage range of acceptable time to be "on red."

Life reminder: People will take as much as you are willing to give. Set those boundaries so you can both win.

MAKE A MATRIX

Take stock of everything that's still on your plate, and create an Eisenhower Matrix as follows: Draw a horizontal line intersecting with a vertical line to show four quadrants. The top two quadrants are important, and the bottom two unimportant. The quadrants on the left are urgent; those on the right are nonurgent.

Name the top-left quadrant (important and urgent) "Do." These are the things you'll focus on for the rest of the season. The top-right quadrant (important and nonurgent) is labeled "Defer." Tasks falling here can be scheduled for later on, perhaps next cycle, or at least after the Do tasks. The bottom-left quadrant (urgent and unimportant) is named "Delegate," showing everything that can be assigned to someone else. Finally, the bottom-right quadrant (unimportant and nonurgent) is your "Delete" category. It may be scary at first, but think about it:

Does this task *truly* need to happen? Is it important *and* time sensitive for this cycle? If not, get rid of it, guilt free, knowing you have other priorities.

CLIENT CASE: HOSTING EVENTS

A large part of Ladaisha's job was to coordinate running events. She loved when she got to lead events in her inner summer, since she found she was naturally a strong communicator with high, runner-friendly energy at that time. When she started cycle syncing, she wondered whether she'd feel a lowered performance in other seasons. Would she feel as confident or energetic being a leader on her period?

What Ladaisha found was that each season helped her with her work in a different way. When she was in her inner winter, she actually felt more grounded, calm, and clear-headed at events (as opposed to that head-in-the-stars feeling in summer). Plus, all the other tasks that go into event planning and leading could be put into a cyclical framework, allowing her strengths to shine no matter when the in-person events took place.

You can't always predict—let alone control—when events are scheduled. The key? Leverage the strengths of the season you'll be in.

SUMMARY

Inspired to Observe, Learn, Create, and Improve?

Manage your energy, not your time: The menstrual cycle mirrors the creative cycle. In inner winter you Observe, determining goals and intentions. In inner spring you Learn, gathering information and crafting a game plan. In inner summer you Create, connecting and collaborating while making big moves. And in inner autumn you Improve, wrapping up loose ends and reviewing results.

Play over perfection: You have a built-in system for holistic productivity at work; you just have to know the signs and how to react to them. Every cycle, you get a chance to look at the big picture, plan out the details, reach the goals, and analyze the results. You'll never be able to perfectly align your cycle to work—that's unrealistic, since life is unpredictable. So play around, find a few habits, and see what sticks.

Your experience above all: When you plan out your work projects with your cycle, you can predict when certain tasks will yield the highest impact. You'll know when you'll be motivated to do certain work and what your strengths will be each week. This cycle may look different from that of your colleagues or friends—that's okay! You're a unique human, remember?

Whether you use your menstrual cycle as your primary guide or use another framework to make your workflow cyclical, you have the power to feel more energized, inspired, and, yes, "productive" at work!

● ● ●

MAP OUT A PROJECT'S CYCLE

Think of one work or creative project on the docket. It should be sizable enough that it'll take at least a few weeks, start to finish.

Project: ....

Write down the goal and the why of this particular project.

Goal: ....

....

Why: ....

....

Brainstorm all the tasks you'd need to do to bring this project to life. (Peek back at the creative cycle if you need help thinking!) Write them all down in any order they come to mind.

Now, place a check mark in the corresponding column for each task's optimal season.

TASK	W	SP	SU	A
	❏	❏	❏	❏
	❏	❏	❏	❏
	❏	❏	❏	❏

THE CYCLE SYNCING HANDBOOK

TASK	W	SP	SU	A
	❏	❏	❏	❏
	❏	❏	❏	❏
	❏	❏	❏	❏
	❏	❏	❏	❏
	❏	❏	❏	❏
	❏	❏	❏	❏
	❏	❏	❏	❏
	❏	❏	❏	❏
	❏	❏	❏	❏

If you're a spreadsheet person, create a digital to-do list showing the tasks organized by season with determined due dates. If you're a visual person, draw a circle and list the four seasons in order around the circle. Place your tasks in the corresponding part of the circle, and check them off as you go.

● ● ●

CHAPTER 7

MOVEMENT AND YOUR CYCLE

* * *

Tendinitis, IT band syndrome, stress fractures... I was riddled with injuries in my early twenties, when sports were my favorite way to spend my time. A new injury was heartbreaking and left me feeling disconnected from my own body.

It was incredibly frustrating to think I was doing all I could to be healthy, just to end up sidelined from my favorite hobbies. I ran hard, I played hard, I strength-trained hard, I stretched hard, I sometimes took a day off.

I decided to train for a marathon and quickly got injured after running just nine miles early in the training calendar. I signed up for a half marathon and struggled through a cobbled-together training plan, then had to cancel due to an emergency surgery weeks before. I registered for event after event, thinking, "If I just push myself hard enough, something will finally click." Nothing clicked. I still felt flat, injured, or burned out.

And then, I lost my period. For over a year, I didn't ovulate or bleed. I knew that was a red flag, but I buried my concern, thinking, "That happens to some athletes; maybe it's just a sign of fitness."

Little did I know that I was very overtrained and undernourished. When you're bombarded with media telling you to train hard every day, that if you're not getting better you're getting worse, it's easy to ignore the whispers from your own body.

After a cross-country move, I ended up living in a cottage in the woods, with no pavement, cell phone service, gym, or even neighbors for miles around. It was a total lifestyle change that scrapped all my old habits and led me to new ones. I got more into trail running and started to notice qualities of running beyond pace or distance. Even if I was slower or didn't go as far, I usually felt far more fulfilled when my body naturally adjusted itself over terrain, season, and my own energy fluctuations. It was freeing.

When wildfires swept through my region that fall, we all kept indoors to avoid the ash falling from the sky. With no treadmill and little energy due to the smoke, I discovered yoga videos on YouTube. For the first time in life, I slowed way down. Even through all my injuries in the years before, I'd pushed through and found some way to keep moving with higher intensity. But as the forest was ablaze and I had nowhere to go, I got on my mat almost every day and started to listen to my body more deeply than ever before. My period and ovulation returned that fall.

After the smoke cleared, I felt renewed with the epiphany that I could balance the fast-paced sports I loved with periods of slower, lower-intensity movement that still made my body feel great. I started using my menstrual cycle to remind myself to take a few days a cycle of honest recovery *and* to allow days to push toward my max. Soon, I ran my first official trail race, a 10 miler, and won my division without training for it. I happily realized that not doing the same workout every day, and instead changing up my routines and ensuring I had times for building and for rest, was working.

I've since run several ultramarathons, successfully avoiding both injury and burnout through all their training cycles. I've climbed a handful of Cascade Volcanoes, trekked to Everest Base Camp, and hiked across the Grand Canyon and back—all energized, without injury, and while having healthy menstrual cycles.

When it comes to training and exercising with intention, nonlinear patterns are what keep me moving happily and healthily. Thankfully, my menstrual cycle gives me daily reminders on how I can feel my best, even while working toward my ambitious athletic goals.

LINEAR MOVEMENT	CYCLICAL MOVEMENT
Running a set number of miles per day at a moderate pace to train for a marathon	Incorporating a mix of slow-paced runs with interval runs, plus rest days, to train for a marathon
Forcing your body to work out hard on days that you feel exhausted or worn out	Enjoying a variety of exercise activities so you can pick and choose which will feel best for your health that day
Following a strict plan without room for changes or improvisation when life gets stressful	Allowing more rest in certain weeks so you can come back stronger the next

WORKOUT WITHOUT BURNOUT

Ever feel totally off when you try to complete your usual workout? You love to run, but you seem to hit a wall every few weeks when your body can't get in the running groove. Or you hit the gym six days a week, but every once in a while you freak out that you can't hit same weight or reps as usual. Maybe some days, your favorite yoga class seems way too slow-paced and boring for you, and other days it's peaceful bliss.

It's unrealistic to expect to feel your absolute best every single day. The good news? You can learn to predict patterns in how you feel when you move, train, and compete.

The number one priority is making sure you're listening to and caring for your body appropriately. Many menstruators think they're not highly active individuals, simply because they're not competitive. You might not be competing at an elite level or have a competitive mindset, but you might still be exercising at a very high level!

Other menstruators tune out signals from their bodies, ignoring signs and symptoms in the name of linear living. This can lead to injury, burnout, stagnation, frustration, or boredom.

Whether you're an all-around athlete, devoted to one sport, or struggling to fit in enough exercise, it's worth collecting data about your cycle to give you a clearer picture around how movement affects your wellness, and it's worth finding cyclical patterns so you can design habits that help you feel your best at all points of your cycle.

Playing with cycle syncing can encourage a variety of movements across a cycle, allowing you to both challenge your body and let it recover to come back stronger. It also teaches you to give yourself grace when you don't perform the same way every day.

WHAT DOES SCIENCE SAY?

I wish I could tell you that there's plenty of conclusive data on how the menstrual cycle influences exercise performance, but there aren't a ton of studies in this realm at the time of this book's publication, and evidence from current research is mixed.

There have been some quality research methods to compare follicular vs. luteal phase performance, and it seems that cyclical fluctuations may play a role in performance. One school of thought is that it seems strength and muscle growth are higher in the follicular phase, when estrogen is high and progesterone is absent. But it's not enough to draw conclusive recommendations for the general public.

Plus, researchers often run into limitations on female exercise science. Some studies don't account for accurately tracking ovulation, and instead count days based off of a 28-day cycle (which most menstruators don't have). Other studies don't allow enough time for participants to restore typical cycles after stopping hormonal birth control or experiencing childbirth. And, so little research has been done on trans people; studies currently focus on cis women (so I unfortunately can't write about the trans experience in this area).

What we do know:

❀ Metabolism speeds up in the luteal phase (after ovulation and before menstruation).

❀ Low energy intake (not enough nutrients) affects hormones in a way that can leave you with frustrating symptoms.

❀ Progesterone is catabolic (it breaks down muscle), and eating enough protein prevents muscle wasting.

❀ Negative cycle-related symptoms (like premenstrual syndrome) can make people *feel* worse, which can lead them not to perform as well.

❀ It's possible to perform your best at any part of the cycle!

Additionally, there are countless anecdotal accounts about how individuals feel and perform at different points of the cycle. Remember the cycle syncing pillar, "Your experience above all"? That's why collecting data as an individual is so important. You might find that your premenstrual symptoms get in the way of performing well, while your friend might hit their best performances in the days before their period.

While science is still developing, I encourage you to focus on your own lived experience, including your athletic goals. Cycle syncing your movement can be beneficial to many menstruators for the way it brings awareness to the body's changes, variety to a training plan, and empowerment in knowing what you need.

MAKE SURE YOU'RE
MOVING ENOUGH FIRST

Hold on! Before you start cycle syncing, there's a prerequisite: getting enough movement to meet health guidelines.

Looking at the Center for Disease Control guidelines on exercise for adults, aim for:

✿ 150 minutes of *moderate-intensity* physical activity per week (that would be 30 minutes a day, 5 days a week) and 2 days of muscle strengthening activity per week

✿ *Or* 75 minutes of *vigorous-intensity* aerobic activity per week and 2 days of muscle strengthening activity per week

(The CDC describes moderate intensity as brisk walking, and vigorous intensity as running/jogging.[4])

Be real with yourself: Are you hitting those benchmarks? If you're not yet getting the minimum amount of recommended exercise, start there! Moving enough is more important than getting into the nitty gritty around your cycle.

MOVEMENT CYCLE MEETS
MENSTRUAL CYCLE

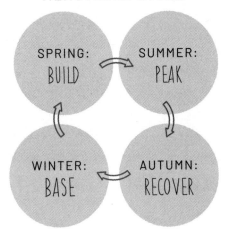

SPRING: BUILD

SUMMER: PEAK

WINTER: BASE

AUTUMN: RECOVER

---

4 US Department of Health and Human Services, "Nutrition and Physical Activity: Current Guidelines," last accessed August 7, 2023, https://health.gov/our-work/nutrition-physical-activity/physical-activity -guidelines/current-guidelines.

THE CYCLE SYNCING HANDBOOK

Unfortunately, cis women in the United States as a group fall far below these guidelines, putting them at higher risk for metabolic disease, bone loss, and muscle loss. They're also less likely to engage in adult sports compared to cis men, and more likely to undereat (which can hurt performance). We need to start with the basics.

Of course, you can use your cycle to start your plan to get enough exercise per week. Perhaps in one inner season, you focus on moderate-intensity exercise, while in the next you add in more vigorous-intensity exercise. Or maybe you plan group exercise classes for when you'll feel most social. You could even switch out your two weekly strength-training sessions with different workouts for each season. You can still have fun with it; the point is that getting *enough* movement each week is the first step to feeling your best.

INNER WINTER: BASE

How you feel during your inner winter depends a lot on how you feel during your period. Although research isn't yet clear on exactly how hormonal fluctuation itself affects athletic performance, we do know that feeling crappy due to symptoms has a negative effect on how you perform. Obviously, if your cramps make you want to curl up on the floor and cry, you are unlikely to hit a 5k personal record!

But no matter what, an active body needs periodic rest. If your period gives you a painful few days, maybe those first few days of your cycle can be your days to focus on rest and recovery. For me personally, I take it easiest the couple days before my period begins. As an endurance athlete, I'm quite active. If I take two intentional days in a row off from any exercise, it's almost always those last two days of my cycle.

So, you've found a time for rest, no matter where exactly you placed it in your training cycle. What comes next? A strong base.

Inner winter is a great time to build a solid foundation for fitness. Just because inner winter is a time of stillness doesn't mean that you have to be *physically* still. (After all, there's skiing!) How can you add more mental stillness to your workouts? Take a break from the headphones and take in the sounds around you. Go to a peaceful natural setting for your workout. Practice following your breath, or try breathing techniques. Think about the clarity and restoration of inner winter and find your way to add a dose of it to your preferred workout.

What happens if you have an athletic event during your period?

❀ Try a menstrual cup or disc. Since they can hold more blood than a tampon, you don't need to find a trashcan, and you can avoid tampon string chafing.

❀ If you choose to use tampons, use an anti-chafe balm to prevent discomfort from the string. Bring a little trash baggie in case you need to change it and carry out trash.

❀ Bring wet wipes to the event.

❀ Avoid tight waistbands. They can aggravate stomach problems, a common period symptom.

❀ If you're nervous about leaks, invest in a pair of period undies.

❀ If you're self-conscious about others potentially noticing, wear a dark, patterned pair of bottoms.

❀ Fuel and hydrate sufficiently. If your stomach gets sensitive, go for bland foods. Watch out for dehydration; it can make any symptoms feel worse.

❀ Allow extra time to use the restroom before the start.

❀ Prep before the event with your personal needs in mind: take your supplements, use a heating pad to calm down cramps, and do whatever you need to do to feel mentally and physically well.

INNER SPRING: BUILD

After you establish a solid fitness base, you can start building on it. Inner spring brings that increase in energy, so harness it by building your fitness!

The curiosity and playfulness powers of inner spring also encourage you to try something new as it pertains to fitness, like that class you've had your eye on, a new sports club, dancing, or a new hiking loop. If you took a step back from higher-intensity movement during your winter, you can start ramping up here. Many menstruators feel happy timing their exercise for midday in their inner spring, due to rising estrogen.

Also, at this time you can plan ahead for the coming week so you can schedule any big workouts or adventures during inner summer.

INNER SUMMER: PEAK

After putting in the work to build, it's time to peak! Inner summer's peaking energy, competitiveness, and daredevil attitude make it an excellent time to push for a personal record.

Testosterone and estrogen peak, giving you motivation, confidence, and energy in your workouts. You might also be attracted to social groups, so run with a pack that can push you or plan a hike with a fun circle of friends. The morning is a great time to work out around ovulation since motivation is high and you have energy to burn. Don't forget to eat and refuel—remember, it's easy to forget your needs when everything is so exciting!

Enjoy your high-intensity interval training (HIIT), heavy lifting, mountain climbing, all the tough challenges—as long as you're feeling up to it.

INNER AUTUMN: RECOVER

After hitting a summit, you need to descend. After hitting maximum speed, a car eventually needs to slow down. Hello, inner autumn: your reminder that you won't see benefits by staying in peak mode forever. You need to tend to your body and build in recovery.

Inner autumn is ideal for tending to anything you typically neglect. Think injury recovery, deep stretches, or those smaller muscle groups you forget about. You know, actually do those things your physical therapist told you to. Inner autumn will create the tendency to turn back inward, so you may prefer working out solo instead of in a group setting. Plus, it's a good time to work through pent-up anger or emotions on your own!

Toward the start of this phase, you may feel similar to the ovulatory time and feel best exercising earlier in the day. As the days pass, you may slip toward gentle evening movement to wind down and support healthy sleep (especially if you experience PMS!).

If you start feeling PMS symptoms, take special care to feel more comfortable. For example, sore breasts might keep you from doing high-intensity jumping exercises; listen to your body's needs and wear extra-supportive clothing.

OVULATION: THE TURNING POINT

Remember that ovulation—the release of an egg from your ovary—is the main event of your menstrual cycle. The time between the start of your period and ovulation is the biological follicular phase. The time between ovulation and the start of your next period is the biological luteal phase.

When it comes to exercise, ovulation is a dividing line:

❋ Metabolism is slower in the follicular phase than during the luteal phase. (That's why you feel hungrier before your period—your metabolism speeds up after ovulation, so you need more calories.)

❋ Basal body temperature is lower in the follicular phase than in your luteal phase (so you won't get as hot while working out).

❋ Approaching ovulation, peaking estrogen and testosterone make many menstruators feel awesome with high energy, endurance, and ambition to reach goals.

❋ The follicular phase is estrogen-dominant, while the luteal phase is progesterone-dominant. Progesterone is catabolic by nature (it breaks down muscle).

Again, researchers aren't entirely sure what that all means in a practical sense (yet!). But it does give us a starting point to optimizing movement throughout our cycle and explains why you feel certain symptoms at different points over the weeks.

PREMENSTRUAL PERFORMANCE

You can absolutely still work out hard in your inner autumn; just be intentional about recovery and nutritional strategies! Note: I'm not a registered dietitian, so I recommend you find an awesome one if you need support in your athletic goals.

The good news is that research so far shows that your VO2 max (the fastest rate at which your body can use oxygen while exercising) and lactate threshold (in simple terms, the point when you start to feel your muscles burn during aerobic exercise) remain static throughout the cycle, so you can still perform your best at any time of your cycle. You just might need to prepare more for exercise in your luteal phase in order to balance out all those extra factors that didn't affect your body in the follicular phase.

Another fact we know from science: in your luteal phase, you'll need an increase in calories, protein, and rest to feel optimal.

If you have an athletic event during your luteal phase, try the following tips:

❀ Prep the day before and the day of your event by hydrating and getting in sodium. Electrolytes will help here.

❀ Prevent premenstrual cramping by making sure you get in magnesium, zinc, and omega-3 fatty acids the week before your period.

❀ If you're prone to menstrual headaches, try getting in foods that are rich in nitric oxide. Foods like beets, pomegranates, watermelon, and spinach can help ease the shift in blood pressure in the luteal phase.

❀ If constipation is an issue, look into magnesium and make sure you're getting enough fiber.

Being in your luteal phase or inner autumn for an athletic event isn't a bad thing! Progesterone has a calming effect on the brain, which can reduce anxiety and help you focus. Your body is more primed to use fat as a fuel source, which is helpful in endurance activities. And, depending on what you're doing, you might even welcome the elevated body temperature. I sure do, when I'm sleeping on a glacier.

INCORPORATING CYCLE SYNCING INTO YOUR EXISTING ROUTINES

If you're a one-sport athlete, consider how you can adapt your sessions over the course of a cycle, making time for base, build, peak, and recovery workouts. You can adjust the lengths of your warm-ups, increase rest time between exercises or workouts, or modify routes, poses, and moves based on your current hormone levels. You can even set your training plans to have building weeks before ovulation and a premenstrual recovery so that training blocks align with your physiology.

If you're a multisport athlete, you might have fun planning different sports for different phases. You can do more higher-intensity or interval sports in the follicular phase, and increase steady-state endurance movement in the luteal phase.

Remember, science isn't yet proving any one-size-fits-all method. So choose what appeals to you: train consistently throughout a cycle, or push more in your follicular phase and not quite as hard or as much in the late luteal phase.

Basically, play around and experiment until you discover what feels sustainable to you. Work out your hardest in the weeks you feel best, and plan recovery time on the days you feel worst.

TWEAK YOUR PLAN

A good training plan in any sport will include periods of recovery here and there. But most exercise science research is done on people with penises. This means that most training plans are linear and don't account for those of us with menstrual cycles. Unless you find a plan or coach who can consider your cycle, you might want to make your own modifications to your routines.

Perhaps your plan includes a certain number of training sessions within one month. You might be able to front-load more than half of the total number of workouts in half your cycle, then have fewer workouts to complete in the second half. Then, even if your workouts are exactly the same, the cadence is a bit different to adjust to your energy.

Let's take running as an example. (Have you been able to tell I run a lot?) When it comes to running, most training plans have a recovery week every third or fourth week. I try to have that week align with the late luteal phase of my cycle, which for me is my late autumn into early winter. It doesn't always perfectly line up, but I feel great knowing that I have two concepts backing me up 1) trusting the training process, 2) knowing I can train by effort instead of by a certain pace or distance. If my pace is slower in my late luteal phase but it feels like the same effort as my faster follicular phase paces, then my body is adjusting for me!

RPE

If you want to start training with your cycle, you don't have to make any drastic changes! RPE—rating of perceived exertion—is a tool you can use to avoid changing any workout plans while accounting for how you feel.

RPE is a quick and easy way to adjust exercise for any lifestyle changes that happen over the course of your cycle. An RPE of 1 is just above a resting effort, at hardly any physical exertion, whereas an RPE of 10 is as hard as you can possibly go, your maximum effort.

You might lift heavier at an RPE of 8 during certain times of your cycle compared to others. In other words, even if the effort feels the same between those two times, you can lift heavier in one at that same perceived intensity. In my running example, an eight-minute mile in my late inner autumn may feel the same RPE as a seven-minute mile in my inner spring.

THE CYCLE SYNCING HANDBOOK

By dedicating an RPE goal for each workout (which is best if decided by someone trained to do so, like a coach or a certified training plan), you can rest assured that you're hitting the training efforts you're supposed to, without changing any metrics.

MAKE OTHER TRAINING ASPECTS CYCLICAL

If you're dedicated to a plan or don't need or want to change your workouts at all based on your cycle, you can sync other factors that relate to movement.

Instead of adapting the *what* of your workouts, you can change the *when, where,* and *with whom.* A few ideas:

❀ Change the time of day at which you work out based on your season.

❀ Switch up your environment: rotate between trails, parks, gyms, fields, or even parts of your home, along with your cycle.

❀ Balance solo training with one-on-one workouts and group meet-ups, depending on how social your season makes you feel.

SLEEP

You already know this, don't you? Adequate sleep is critical for athletic performance and recovery (plus general health and feeling well, of course). Getting enough sleep helps you rebuild muscle, replenishes energy, regulates stress hormones (which affect sex hormones downstream), and helps your mental game.

Some menstruators find sleep disturbances related to their cycle, most commonly just before the start of menstruation and the days of the period itself. Some people also notice disturbances in the luteal phase, when basal body temperature rises.

Is your cycle affecting your sleep? See if you're missing one of these tips:

❀ Limit your caffeine after noon (at the latest).

❀ Set a tech curfew for at least two hours before bedtime (use that DND mode).

❀ Maintain a consistent bedtime every night.

❀ Get in that daily exercise.

❀ Manage your light exposure; keep your bedroom dark and avoid glaring light from phones or other electronics.

❀ Have a pre-sleep routine to mentally get ready for bed.

❀ Keep your bedroom cool.

- ❀ Invest in a great pillow and mattress (my nice pillow changed my life and hugely helped my chronic neck pain).
- ❀ Use reliable, comfortable period products. I love period panties on my first couple nights of flow, even if I'm using my cup, too. In my experience, what wakes me up is the thought that I'm leaking on the sheets!

THE ADVENTURE CYCLE

Got an adventurous spirit? Me too. I love getting in the wilderness to chase big goals. What I've noticed (and absolutely adore) is that a true adventure is also cyclical.

First, you have to dream it. One day, you get a teeny nudge in your brain to *do the thing.* You see someone complete a 50-mile backcountry run, or a friend spends a month kite boarding across Greenland, or your cousin circumnavigates the Channel Islands in a sea kayak, or your neighbor climbs a Himalayan peak. You realize *you* want to, need to, do something big and adventurous too. This is the inner winter phase: a time to get clarity on your adventure dream and make sure it matters to you.

Then, you need to plan it. This inner spring season can take weeks or months, depending on the expedition. You research routes and put your strategizing brain to work. You make packing lists, reach out to adventure partners, seek out funding, and ask others who have done similar adventures for advice. You gobble up all you can to set yourself up for success.

Heck yes, it's time to do it! It's your inner summer, the season to get out there and live your best adventure. You prepared for this, so you feel confident and joyous, like you were made to be outside in the wild. You can live in full bloom and full flow, entirely engaged in the adventure at hand and working smoothly with your team if you have one. And in the blink of an eye, you're home!

Finally, for closure, you reflect on the adventure. An expedition—heck, even a single backcountry ski day—isn't complete without an intentional debrief. You analyze your journey, determine what went well and what could be improved, laugh at the extra gear you didn't need, and cry thinking back to what you wish you brought instead. You celebrate your accomplishments and share your adventure story with the world.

CLIENT CASE: GOING WITH THE FLOW

Skyler's a talented white-water kayaker who lives in British Columbia. She noticed that some days she felt on top of her game, and other days she couldn't figure out why she felt anxious, annoyed, or simply fatigued on the water. The inconsistency frustrated her to no end—*before* she noticed cyclical patterns.

As she learned to track and chart her cycles, she dug into cycle syncing, too. That's when it became clear to her: The changes weren't inconsistent, they were cyclical. She felt a little "spacey" and less excited about paddling in her inner winter, loved practicing drills and tricks in her inner spring, felt bravest in her inner summer, and felt self-critical (and hungrier) in inner autumn. A classic case of cyclical patterns.

Once she noticed the cyclical nature of her experiences, Skyler could prepare for paddling throughout her cycle. She starting scheduling her biggest pushes for her inner summer and took extra care to fuel more and sleep more premenstrually, especially before races and big runs. Even just knowing that her self-esteem tends to drop in her inner autumn helped—she had a reason that she felt off, and then she could challenge her inner critic.

I've connected with a handful of river runners who note their cycles in their sport:

- ❀ "I never try to run a harder river than normal when I'm premenstrual." —Tish
- ❀ "I personally find bleeding on river trips extremely liberating. I even look forward to having my period on the river." —Elliot
- ❀ "I started my period the morning of Lava [the biggest rapid on the Grand Canyon]. It gave me so much confidence somehow." —Cate

As a former river guide, I was thrilled to see more boaters noticing and embracing their cycles. I even wrote an entire 1,500-word blog post on how to sync your cycle as a whitewater boater. (It's actually one of my most popular blog posts ever.)

It goes beyond the actual river (or field, or trail, or mountain). You might find that gear repair and maintenance is best for inner autumn, while journaling your experiences comes most easily in inner winter.

No matter your sport, can you identify the powers of, challenges of, and ways to embrace each season?

SUMMARY

You can incorporate movement that honors your base, build, peak, and recover phases.

Manage your energy, not your time: If you feel less pep in your step during a certain season (for many of us, that's inner autumn into inner winter), you don't need to totally step away from exercise or your training goals. Instead, maybe you need to sleep more (or sleep better) to feel refreshed, fuel more (especially protein after workouts and carbs before them), or space out your harder training sessions, scheduling your maintenance instead of build weeks then.

Play over perfection: Even if you feel differently in each phase, you're still capable of performing your best at any point of the cycle. Don't stress if you can't change much of your training around your cycle! Focusing on other aspects of cycle syncing can still help.

Your experience above all: Some people love working out on their period; others detest it. As long as you're getting enough exercise, you're not over-training or underfueling, and you're enjoying movement, then there's no right or wrong way to exercise cyclically.

Athletes who are deeply connected to their bodies perform better in their bodies. By increasing your knowledge and empowerment around your menstrual cycle, you can get an edge on your goals while respecting your biology. Win-win!

● ● ●

CYCLICAL WORKOUT LOG

For the next full cycle, log how you feel every time you intentionally exercise. Rate each workout with perceived exertion (see the RPE section on page 98) and describe how you felt. Did you adjust the plan due to your cycle? Did you want to switch up the when, where, or with whom?

DATE	WORKOUT TYPE	INNER SEASON	RPE 1-10	NOTES

● ● ●

CHAPTER 8

FOOD AND YOUR CYCLE

• • •

On my twenty-first birthday, the bone doctor diagnosed me with "the worst metatarsal stress fracture he's ever seen." He sternly added that I wasn't eating properly to heal the injury. The strict rigidity of my diet would slow my healing and keep me from playing the sports I loved. But I had no clue on how to best fuel myself.

Linear eating dominated my nutrition in those years, so much so that I developed some disordered eating patterns. I had the same breakfast every day (which I thought was reasonable, but in hindsight was way too small for my active lifestyle). I'd think, "I already ate a yogurt today, so now I have to find a different snack" and "I need to have protein or else that workout was useless." If I let myself slip from my rigid eating routines, I'd have the weekend "F it!" attitude and end up eating a lot of food that wasn't even tasty, leaving me uncomfortable and thinking I had no willpower. Not to mention, meals were *so* boring.

After adopting my puppy Kudo a few years into those unhealthy habits, my routine was shaken up. I had to move apartments, take my sweet pup out to pee in the middle of the night, go straight home from work to give him a walk, and watch him constantly to make sure he wasn't eating any shoelaces. It was exhausting.

Being a new dog mom quickly took its toll. On my twenty-fourth birthday, I lied on the couch and quietly cried, more fatigued than I'd ever been before. I couldn't keep up with the lifestyle of caring for a puppy, maintaining all my hobbies, and working when I wasn't getting enough energy (or pleasure) from food. I did a bit of googling, realized I had orthorexic tendencies (research orthorexia if my story is relatable), and started listening to a podcast by a registered dietitian. That's when I learned about intuitive eating, and my healing finally began.

True intuitive eating (in the way authors and nutrition experts Elyse Resch and Evelyn Tribole teach it) shook me out of my linear, unhelpful eating patterns. It took months, but I started to note how my taste preferences changed over days, weeks, and months. I noticed that some days, I'd feel fuller more quickly, and other times I'd need more food to feel satiated. I started to find immense pleasure in trying new foods, buying foods I used to restrict, keeping a (very tiny) garden, and avoiding overthinking around nutrition, instead allowing my intuition and body to tell me what I needed.

Around that time, I dove into cycle syncing myself and found that living more cyclically with food gave me the nutrients, energy, flexibility, and joy around nutrition that I'd been missing in college. I could finally keep up with my beautiful Kudo through mountain walks and shoelace nibbling.

Tuning into my cycle had many parallels with tuning into my hunger, and the two worked in tandem to help me feel energized and nourished all cycle long. I haven't looked back.

LINEAR EATING	CYCLICAL EATING
Following a meal plan that has you eat the same foods and meals every day	Changing up the menu day to day or week to week to allow for a variety of nutrients
Eating the same portion size all cycle long, no matter your hunger levels	Being mindful to get more calories premenstrually, increasing protein when necessary and consuming foods to help with PMS and period symptoms when needed
Forcing yourself into a strict diet plan that you can only manage in the short term before giving up	Eliminating the word "guilt" around food, and experimenting with sustainable methods to reach health goals

PLAY WITH YOUR FOOD

It's simple—and fun—to incorporate different foods in each phase of your menstrual cycle, and there's no need to be restrictive or perfect! Rather, when you're grocery shopping for the coming week, shop for the foods that help you feel your best in your coming season.

The benefit of eating with your cycle in mind is that you'll naturally give your body a variety of nutritious foods to support your energy and hormone health. And that helps on the long road: When you make significant health changes, it takes about three months for the results to show up in your reproductive system (which is why some people looking to become pregnant hope to optimize the health of their eggs by making changes a few months before trying to conceive). That means in a few months, you can decrease PMS symptoms or period pain.

Your ovaries and uterus are doing different things at different times, and this gives you a delicious chance to honor their needs. Plus, over the course of a cycle, your metabolism, digestion, blood sugar response, and micronutrient levels change! As you explore, remember to honor your circadian rhythm, too, by eating at regular intervals and not letting yourself get too hungry, or worse, hangry.

DIPPING YOUR TOE IN

You never have to go all-in with cycle syncing. I hope that's clear by now! Especially when it comes to food, there are barriers all over the place. In the United States, it's often cheaper to buy fast food than quality produce. We live in hustle culture, where it's hard even to make time to sit and eat. Food can be dang expensive, whether you're cooking yourself or eating out!

A few ideas to try eating cyclically without pulling out your hair:

- ❀ **Start with just one element, like produce.** As you get accustomed to rotating foods with your cycle, go with one food group at a time. Fruits and veggies are a wonderful place to start.

- ❀ **Create season-specific shopping lists.** As you read this chapter, take notes on what foods you want to try eating in each season. Separate them and save a copy on your phone so you always know what to stock up on at the store based on what season you're in.

- ❀ **Batch cook whenever you can.** At the start of a season, I love cooking a huge batch of grains that'll last almost a week in the fridge. A lot of inner autumn and inner winter meals are freezer friendly, so cook extra whenever you have more energy.

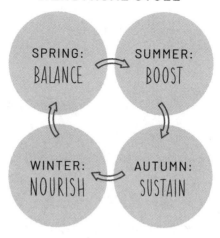

FOOD CYCLE MEETS MENSTRUAL CYCLE

SPRING:
BALANCE

SUMMER:
BOOST

WINTER:
NOURISH

AUTUMN:
SUSTAIN

INNER WINTER: NOURISH

What foods come to mind when you think of a hearty winter meal? Probably warm, comforting, nourishing foods that make you want to curl up by the fireplace with a good book. You might crave that same cozy feeling during your period.

Inflammation causes pain, which people who experience painful periods know all too well. Even if it's not exactly pain, many other menstruators experience discomfort in some way at some time during their period. And, after the body sheds its uterine lining, nutrition is a way to build back those iron stores and B vitamins lost through bleeding. In your inner winter, food can serve a few purposes: reduce inflammation, maximize comfort, and restore micronutrients.

When you approach inner winter meals, think "warmth and replenishment." Hot, hearty meals like soups, stews and curries, plus high-fiber carbs can be both mentally grounding and physically nourishing. Warming foods are usually gentler on the stomach (since the stomach is already warm, thanks to your core temperature), which might ease cramps, too. Have fun incorporating anti-inflammatory spices for inner winter, like cinnamon, ginger, turmeric, cardamom, cumin, and cayenne.

Iron, vitamins C and B12, omega-3 fatty acids, iodine, and zinc all support healthy periods. Are you getting those from your food now, or can you incorporate more?

Some great additions to your inner winter menu:

- ❋ Beets (good source of iron; help with bloating)
- ❋ Watermelon (hydrating; helps with water retention)
- ❋ Mushrooms (B vitamins for energy)
- ❋ Dark chocolate (good source of magnesium, but does it need an excuse?)
- ❋ Pumpkin seeds (high in zinc)
- ❋ Seaweed, like kelp (good source of iron, iodine, and magnesium)

INNER SPRING: BALANCE

When inner winter turns into inner spring, what types of food tend to pop up? Usually, they're lighter and brighter than winter meals, plates that make you want to sit outside for a picnic amid the new daffodils. You might gravitate more toward these foods in your *inner* spring, too.

Your spring intention is to nourish your fertility and metabolize estrogen that's starting to build up. Your menstrual cycle wants your body to start preparing to release an egg, so you can use food as a tool to promote healthy ovulation.

Consider light, fresh, and colorful foods as you welcome inner spring. You might incorporate light grains, fresh or fermented veggies, citrus, and nuts and seeds. You can play with cooling herbs like peppermint, basil, or dill. Your gut and liver will thank you for eating foods that help process estrogen, like cruciferous veggies and flaxseed. Steaming and sautéing are excellent cooking methods in this season.

You might notice a decrease in appetite or feel like you can get by on less food, since estrogen regulates your brain's hunger signals. Remember, biology wants you out and about looking for a mate, not at home cooking. Plus, your metabolism is lower here compared to after ovulation. Because of that, you might not think about food as much, so make an effort to remember to fuel adequately.

Options to add to your spring menu:

- ❋ Broccoli (supports healthy metabolism of estrogen)
- ❋ Avocado (good source of fat)
- ❋ Cashews (rich in fiber and fat)

THE CYCLE SYNCING HANDBOOK

* Green peas (vitamins C, E, and zinc)
* Oats (carbs and fiber)
* Artichoke (antioxidant-rich, and an alleged aphrodisiac!)

INNER SUMMER: BOOST

When the heat of summer strikes, what do you crave to cool you off? A smoothie, fresh fruit, or a salad straight from the garden? Inner summer may be the time you're most likely to grab those light, fresh, cooling foods that energize you.

Inner summer's focus is to support energy levels and estrogen detoxification. You'll ovulate in this season, so nutrition can help you manage the buildup of estrogen beforehand and the swing in hormones afterward.

It's a great time for berries and leafy greens. You might be satisfied with less, so lighter grains can feel good here, like quinoa and corn. Restock those cruciferous veggies that you enjoyed during inner spring to keep processing that estrogen, and keep those cooling herbs and spices coming. You might like raw foods more than usual, plus there's the perk of not spending as much time cooking if you choose raw. Otherwise, you might like juices and steamed meals.

Just like in inner spring, you may be fertile, so nature decreases your appetite so you can focus on being out in the world. You might have to remind yourself to eat, especially when you're caught up in all the inner summer fun. It's easy to get distracted when you're accomplishing so much!

A few ideas to add to your inner summer grocery list:
* Corn (lighter grain, B vitamins)
* Pecans (protein, fat, and fiber)
* Brussels sprouts (estrogen detoxification)
* Raspberries (antioxidants)
* Coconut (nutritious fat)
* Asparagus (folic acid, potassium)

INNER AUTUMN: SUSTAIN

As you think about the shift into autumn, imagine the foods you start craving. Many menstruators seek out warm, hearty meals that boost their mood and contain nutrients. Think of a love-filled Friendsgiving dinner! This is your inner autumn's nutrition vibe.

Inner autumn wants to help you build up nutrients to prepare you for your upcoming period, as well as boost your premenstrual mood and optimize sleep with the help of feel-good foods. Loading up on nutrients now can make your period feel better, and supporting progesterone can help ease PMS symptoms.

Imagine a fall harvest of hearty, filling foods to help you prepare for inner winter, like root vegetables and potatoes, whole grains, brown rice, leafy greens, and beans. Make sure you get your fill of foods with magnesium (dark chocolate, anyone?), omega-3 fatty acids, and vitamins D and B6. B vitamins can support energy and help with pesky premenstrual sugar cravings. A dash of warming herbs and spices is lovely here, too. You might try baking and roasting more often in your inner autumn.

A lot of menstruators deal with slower digestion—read, constipation—in this phase. Fiber-rich foods will lead to better poops. More on that in a minute.

Your metabolism speeds up in the luteal phase, and your brain encourages you to stay home and get in food just in case you could be pregnant (again, even if that's not possible). If you get cravings or are extra hungry in this season, honor that! Trying to fight your biology will only make it more frustrating. You need more calories and more nutrients than you did when you were fertile, and that's okay. It's all a part of the cycle.

Foods to work in to your inner autumn meals:

- ❀ Yams (potassium, complex carb)
- ❀ Apples (fiber, hydration)
- ❀ Ginger (helps with nausea, comforting)
- ❀ Cauliflower (good source of choline; supports mood and metabolism)
- ❀ Sunflower seeds (vitamin E, might support healthy progesterone levels)
- ❀ Squash (tons of vitamins, grounding)

PMS-FIGHTING FOODS

PMS is your body's way of telling you something isn't quite right. You might have too much stress, a hormone imbalance, or nutritional deficiency. This makes annoying symptoms pop up in the days or weeks before your next period.

Tackling PMS is very individual, and of course I'd recommend working with a healthcare provider to make that time of the cycle happier and healthier. But as you experiment with cycle syncing to see what effect it has, consider these nutrition tweaks for the premenstrual days.

CRUCIFEROUS VEGGIES

Why: High estrogen levels can lead to rough PMS symptoms. Cruciferous veggies help your body detoxify estrogen.

Try: Broccoli, brussels sprouts, bok choy, cauliflower, cabbage

CITRUS FRUITS

Why: Healthy levels of progesterone can help prevent PMS. Citrus contains vitamin C, which can boost progesterone.

Try: Oranges, grapefruit, lemon

OMEGA- 3 FATTY ACIDS

Why: Increasing omega-3 (and decreasing omega-6) intake can help decrease inflammation.

Try: Oily fish (like salmon, mackerel, and sardines), cod liver oil, flax seeds, chia seeds, walnuts

COMPLEX CARBOHYDRATES

Why: Unlike simple carbs, complex carbs gradually enter the bloodstream to help stabilize blood sugar. (Added bonus: fiber!)

Try: Sweet potatoes, lentils, squash, barley, quinoa, beans

WHEN YOU GET CRAVINGS

Everybody gets cravings from time to time. But many people try to either stifle those cravings or go all in on giving into the craving with less nutritious options than they'd like.

Instead, think of cravings as a signal from your body telling you what it needs in that moment, then take a mindful moment to find a meal or snack that will satisfy the craving without making you crash shortly afterward.

By the way—there's no shame in giving in to your cravings! Mindfully enjoy whatever food you choose to eat. Wellness comes from taking care of yourself over time, not the occasional indulgence in the moment.

SWEET CRAVINGS

Craving the cake, cookies, and honey-lavender lattes? Your body actually wants *energy*, and since sugar gives it the quickest hit, you feel that sweet tooth appear.

Try lessening the urge with rice, honey, fruit, sweet potatoes, cacao, and complex carbs. And make sure you're getting enough magnesium in your diet. Fifty percent of people are deficient!

SALTY CRAVINGS

Can't get enough salt? You might be dehydrated or you could be stressed out. Get the salt craving satisfied with dry-roasted nuts, kale or seaweed chips, homemade sweet potato chips, or eggs.

Use this as a reminder to check in with your stress levels! When your adrenals are taxed, it affects how you eat.

SOUR CRAVINGS

Looking for an acidic bite? Your body might need some digestive support. Try satisfying sour cravings with fermented foods like sauerkraut and Greek yogurt, citrus fruits, kombucha, or lemon water.

Regularly fitting acidic foods into your diet helps keep your stomach acid levels balanced, which is, of course, a key to healthy digestion.

BITTER CRAVINGS

Although less common than sweet cravings, bitter cravings happen and let you know that you could use some antioxidants. Plus, some people crave bitter foods when they're feeling down, so it's worth checking your mood!

Consider having bitter foods like dark chocolate, cacao, dandelion greens, or other leafy greens.

You might also try ingesting digestive bitters before a meal.

WHEN YOU'RE HANGRY

You know when you don't even care what's on the table, but you want all the food *now*? That's your blood sugar getting out of whack. Prevent the crash before it happens by having a meal or snack every two to four hours. Once you feel a twinge of hunger, have a snack to satisfy it.

When you do get hangry, make sure whatever you choose has a mix of carbohydrate, fat, and protein so you get a well-rounded meal. It helps to keep quick-cooking food prepared in the fridge for a quick fix—and your late inner summer and early inner autumn are a great time to prepare that.

Remember Your Inner Season Tracker (see page 19)? That's a great spot to note any cravings or hanger that pop up in your cycle!

THE DEAL WITH PERIOD POOPS

We've all been there. You feel like you can't go for days, but then your period arrives and it's a totally different story.

In the follicular phase, estrogen is the dominant player, encouraging smooth muscle contractions in your digestive tract to keep things moving efficiently. But the dominant hormone of the luteal phase is progesterone, produced only after ovulation. It has muscle relaxant qualities, which makes it harder for your bowels to contract in the way that leads to bowel movement, so digestion slows down in the luteal phase. Progesterone levels plummet when your period begins. Suddenly, the constipating effect of progesterone disappears, and what's left inside you might come out quickly and loosely.

(Another reason? When uterine contractions increase on your period, bowel contractions can increase, too, adding to the period poop madness.)

So, what can you do?

1. Manage your stress. High cortisol (stress hormone) levels lead to more inflammation, leading to more symptoms downstream.

2. Enjoy anti-inflammatory foods. Those omega-3s, fruits, veggies, nuts and seeds, and whole grains are here to help!

3. Keep an eye on your gut health. You obviously want great digestion all cycle long, not just during your period. If you're not pooping at least once a day or you're having regular diarrhea, you might want to dig into what's going on in your gut by chatting with a healthcare provider.

CLIENT CASES: HOW THEY MAKE FOOD WORK FOR THEIR CYCLES

Nutrition is extremely individual, so I love chatting with others who have tweaked their cyclical strategies to create delicious moments in every phase.

❀ Davida's a triathlete who wanted on-the-go homemade snacks aligned with her cycle. Because she is a fellow endurance athlete who loves making her own snacks and hates the energy gels that many races provide, I encouraged her to make different energy balls for different phases. Her favorite is the "spring ball," formed by freezing a mixture of oats, flax seeds, pumpkin seeds, cashew butter, craisins, maple syrup, and chocolate chips. You can vary the ingredients depending on your season, turn them into bars, or even drizzle melted chocolate over them!

❀ Noel doesn't change her ingredients or shopping lists by season, but she does cook and prepare differently across her cycle. She sets aside time in her inner autumn to batch cook a *lot* of food that she can freeze and use in inner winter. She plans a grilling day for her inner summer so she can cook outdoors. And, she tells me that she splurges on her favorite latte in town just once a cycle, on Day 1. This gives her a little treat to look forward to when she gets her period.

❀ Alma's a parent and prefers cooking food that both she and her children will enjoy. Whenever possible, she sneaks in the nutrients she wants to support her inner season: roasted beet chips for her winter, carrot morning glory muffins for her spring, bright berry smoothies for her summer, and cauliflower crust pizza in her autumn. Find subtle shifts in your recipes so you can swap out ingredients by season.

What will you give a taste next cycle?

SUMMARY

Every cycle's a chance to nourish, balance, boost, and sustain your nutrition.

Manage your energy, not your time: Food is energy. It's what fuels you to go out and do big things in the world. Pay special attention to how your food energizes you (or doesn't) in each phase. Consider why you have certain cravings, whether your meals can ease period symptoms, and what ingredients would be simple to swap around each season. There's no need to micromanage your meals, but finding patterns is eye opening.

Play over perfection: Nutrition is so individualized that you can't copy someone else's food habits entirely. Fad diets and rigid meal plans are unlikely to help you feel your best for a long time. Instead, experiment each cycle to gather data on what works for you.

Your experience above all: Maybe this chapter doesn't resonate with you at all. That's okay! I'm not here to tell you how to eat. If this does inspire you, pick and choose which pieces align with your vision and leave the rest—just like when you're shopping at the grocery store.

Whether you eat with Earth's seasons, plant your own garden, eat out for lunch every day or construct an entire meal plan for each inner season, cyclical eating can keep you inspired and satisfied in the kitchen.

● ● ●

BUILD-A-BOWL TOOL

In a rut and need an easy way to practice cycle syncing *and* ensure you get a quality, satiating meal? Use this build-a-bowl chart to help you construct a simple yet tasty meal no matter what season you're in.

Choose your season's column, then work your way down the categories, picking at least one ingredient from each row.

	INNER WINTER	INNER SPRING	INNER SUMMER	INNER AUTUMN
GRAINS	Buckwheat, rice	Barley, oats	Corn, quinoa	Brown rice, millet
VEGGIES	Beets, kale, kelp, mushrooms	Artichokes, broccoli, carrots, rhubarb, string beans, zucchinis	Asparagus, bell peppers, brussels sprouts, chard, eggplants, spinach, tomatoes	Cabbage, cauliflower, cucumber, garlic, ginger, onion, pumpkin, radish, squash, yam
FRUITS	Berries, grapes, watermelon	Avocado, grapefruit, lemon, lime, orange, plum	Apricots, melons, coconuts, figs, guavas, berries	Apples, dates, peaches, pears, raisins
MEAT/ LEGUMES	Duck, pork, liver, lentils	Chicken, eggs, lentils	Lamb, chickpeas	Beef, turkey, kidney beans

	INNER WINTER	INNER SPRING	INNER SUMMER	INNER AUTUMN
NUTS/ SEEDS	Sesame seeds, sunflower seeds	Brazil nuts, cashew, flax seeds, pumpkin seeds	Almonds, flax seeds, pumpkin seeds, pecans	Pine nuts, walnut, sesame seeds, sunflower seeds
SIDES	Miso, decaf tea, tamari, salt	Vinegar, sauerkraut, pickles, olives	Coffee, turmeric, chocolate	Peppermint, bone broth

What are some other ingredients you love or crave in these seasons? Write them below:

_____

_____

_____

Plan out a bowl that sounds yummy for each season:

My inner winter bowl: _____

_____

My inner spring bowl: _____

_____

My inner summer bowl: _____

_____

My inner autumn bowl: _____

_____

● ● ●

CHAPTER 9

RELATIONSHIPS AND YOUR CYCLE

• • •

Without my encounter with a life-threatening experience, I'm not sure I would've ever come to realize the power of my cycle. The experience led me to revolutionize my relationship with myself and in the world. Get cozy; it's story time.

I got a copper intrauterine device (IUD) inserted for birth control in college. For several years, I reaped the benefits of the IUD. As the rest of my friends set alarm reminders on their phones to take the pill, I sat back and relaxed, knowing my birth control required no reminders, no maintenance, and no worries.

Fast forward more than three years later. I had lost my period for most of that past year and had finally started getting it regularly for a few months. When I started spotting a week after my last period, I assumed it was just my body getting used to its cycle again. Soon, I started to feel strange, intense cramps that lasted just a minute or two a day. Again, I shrugged it off as my body getting back on track after missing my period for so long. I went about my life as usual, despite the on-and-off pain and bleeding.

A few days later, the cramping began to attack more frequently. Having never before experienced a urinary tract infection (UTI) but having heard how horrible they feel, I figured I should get checked for one. I went to an urgent care clinic, where they took my urine. Several minutes later, a doctor entered the room to tell me I simply had an inflamed urethra. I hobbled out of the clinic, pain-fighting prescription in hand.

But after starting the medicine, the pain intensified and continued to do so throughout the night, until I was writhing in pain on my living room floor. I knew I wouldn't be able to sleep in that state. But when I started vomiting, I knew it was more serious than I'd thought. I rushed to the only urgent care that was open at that late hour, where the nurses repeated what the first clinic had done, except they also gave me a pregnancy test.

Shockingly, the test came back positive. I was supposedly pregnant, even with an IUD that was highly effective at preventing just that. They told me they'd already called the emergency room across the street, and that I had to go for an ultrasound and a blood test right away.

The ER staff brought me into a room immediately and hooked me up to what felt like a hundred sensors and cords, including an IV of morphine, which gave me an escape from the stabbing pain as the next few hours slowly passed. Finally, the doctor confirmed the results: my ultrasound revealed an ectopic pregnancy in my right fallopian tube.

An IUD does not *cause* an ectopic pregnancy, but in the ridiculously tiny like-lihood that the IUD fails to prevent pregnancy, there is a higher risk of it being ectopic. Mine had failed. I was part of that sad statistic.

I sat in disbelief, waiting for the specialist who'd been called in. He cut to the chase. I would need surgery. As soon as possible. Even though my preg-nancy hormone levels were low and the pregnancy was extremely early, I had enough internal bleeding that emergency surgery was the only option. Best-case scenario, they'd remove the blood and mass. Worst case, my tube would rupture and I'd need it entirely removed. I went under anesthesia while hoping for the best.

The next thing I knew, I was in a quiet maternity ward. A nurse greeted me. I asked her how it went, thinking and hoping it was the best-case scenario. I was stunned when the nurse replied, "They removed the tube; it had ruptured. There was a lot of blood in there." My shock continued: How could a healthy 24 year old unknowingly be pregnant while on birth control *and* lose a whole tube?

Physically, the recovery was uncomfortable, but the mental effects were far worse. I had to struggle with feeling like a stranger to my body, with the misdi-agnosis from the first clinic, with the fact that I no longer had birth control, and with major anxiety that my body could backfire again with no warning. I tried to figure out what birth control method to try next, when I couldn't trust the most effective form any longer.

Thankfully, my slow-healing process led me to learning the Fertility Awareness Method (FAM) for birth control. This type of birth control involves observing and recording your fertility signs, like basal body temperature and cervical mucus changes, in order to determine days of fertility. (This isn't the rhythm method, which simply counts days and involves guessing when you're fertile, which obviously isn't reliable.)

A whole world opened up for me; I *could* interpret signs from my body and use them to make informed decisions. I could track patterns that gave insightful data into my health and hormones. I didn't need to be anxious about every little twinge in my pelvis, since I now knew what was normal and what was not. I dove into every resource I could to educate myself about my body and reproductive system, which is what led me to train as a birth and fertility doula and become a fertility awareness instructor. My traumatic experience first led me to infinitely deepen my relationship to my own body, then to a passion for helping others interpret *their* bodies.

These discoveries of fertility awareness, cycle syncing, and becoming a business owner concurrently launched me into a whole personal era of self-growth. I was learning to understand my body and purpose, but I wanted to understand my *relationships* better, too.

What parts of my personality could I claim as strengths? Where were my blind spots in relationships? Where did I fit on the introversion–extraversion dichotomy? I thought about it for months, and constantly went back and forth.

Turns out, everything varies with my cycle. One example? I'm more extraverted during my inner spring and summer than during my autumn and winter. Although I always love having social engagements scattered throughout my calendar, scheduling the big or important ones during my inner summer typically enhances my experience, while attending the same event in inner winter might leave me a little spacey or tired. I'm thrilled to network and go to new places during my inner spring, whereas during my inner fall I have a bit less energy and patience for social obligations.

If you relate to feeling like a social butterfly some days and like a hermit on others, or if you wonder why you're more interested in sex and intimacy at seemingly random times, or if you just want to feel more harmony across your relationships to others and yourself... this chapter's for you.

LINEAR RELATIONSHIPS	CYCLICAL RELATIONSHIPS
Forcing yourself to show up to planned engagements, even if you're not excited for them	Accepting that some days you're more socially motivated than others, and planning around them
Sticking to the same old date night every time	Experimenting with new ways to deepen your connection with your partner based on your energy fluctuations
Silently dealing with the annoying habits of loved ones, which makes you dread spending time with them	Confidently setting boundaries with others based on your current needs

RELATIONSHIP CYCLE MEETS MENSTRUAL CYCLE

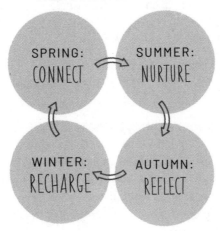

SPRING:
CONNECT

SUMMER:
NURTURE

WINTER:
RECHARGE

AUTUMN:
REFLECT

INNER WINTER: RECHARGE

Ever feel like bailing on happy hour, ignoring all those text messages "until tomorrow," and curling up on the couch with a good book instead?

In your inner winter, you may be very introspective and intuitive, so you could find yourself wanting to spend your free time alone, doing relaxing activities that may be more grounding, quiet, reflective, or meditative. You might choose to catch up on books or movies, journaling or organizing recent photos, or scheduling a long call with a faraway friend.

THE CYCLE SYNCING HANDBOOK

As I hope you know by now: It's totally more than okay for you to let your loved ones know that you need space to recharge! In fact, this is the prime time to nurture the relationship you have with *yourself* by prioritizing self-care and reflection.

ROMANTIC RELATIONSHIPS

Whether you're single, dating, or in a long-term relationship, remember that inner winter typically leads you to seek calmer, more grounding plans. Think of it as a time to nurture each other and restore the love in your relationship.

Syncing your dates for the inner winter season:

❀ **Classic date:** See a light-hearted movie! Simple comedy or rom-com suggested. Extra points for a drive-in theater where you can get extra cozy in your own space.

❀ **At-home date:** Give each other massages. Make your home spa-like with candles, soft music, and scented oils.

❀ **Date with a mindful cycle twist:** On your period, you're more connected to water and fluidity. So, head somewhere with calm water. Think a picnic by the river or an easy canoe or kayak paddle session.

If you're in a romantic relationship, think of quiet, comfortable time together. A light-hearted movie on the sofa, a massage with scented oils, or a relaxing dinner by the lake could feel great here.

Currently single? Avoid going on a date with somebody new. Instead, use this week just for yourself, and treat yourself to something nice during your solo time. Foster that strong connection to yourself before you reemerge into the outer world.

SEX AND INTIMACY

When your period arrives, sex hormones drop to their lowest levels of the cycle. Your cervix sits lower in your pelvis, which means a partner might feel it more easily or you might have more sensation there.

Some people feel disinterested in sex during this phase as a result. At the same time, the pressure of the uterus on the pelvic floor can feel pleasurable for others. Period sex is very individual: some love it, others do without!

Experiment to see what *you* like during your period. Some menstruators have high desire and others none; some have period pain and don't want anyone to touch them, while others feel a reawakening of their sexuality and increased body awareness after the release of premenstrual tension.

Remember, there are plenty of types of sex, not just vaginal penetration, so if that doesn't sound fun to you, you can explore other options. You may even crave solo sex at this time.

If you're concerned about blood, lay down a towel or designate a blanket you can use during period sex and wash afterward. Menstrual discs are a fantastic option; they're similar to menstrual cups but can be used during intercourse.

Please note that blood is *not* a good lubricant! In fact, it's drying. So don't fear the lube in this phase (or any phase).

SETTING HEALTHY BOUNDARIES

Whether it's with yourself, your friends, or your coworkers, protect inner winter's energy by identifying your needs in that phase and setting appropriate limits.

A few boundaries my clients have set during inner winter:

- ❀ Uninstalling social media for a few days
- ❀ Not accepting last-minute meetings
- ❀ Changing email signatures to allow for longer response time
- ❀ Scheduling a nonnegotiable solo hike to reconnect with themselves
- ❀ Setting "do not disturb mode" on their phone after 6 p.m.

INNER SPRING: CONNECT

For many people, noticing the first signs of spring after a long, dark winter is thrilling and hopeful. It can feel the same in your body!

The arrival of inner spring leads many menstruators to feel reenergized and inspired. You'll be drawn to new experiences and more busy, social atmospheres. If you're planning to begin a new habit or hobby, try to start it here. You'll also be more extroverted, so plan nights out with friends or dates this week. It's a fun time to reconnect with your loved ones and plan exciting activities together!

The more cycles you intentionally observe and record, the more patterns you'll pick up. You might find that it's a particular day that brings a fresh spring (for me, Cycle Day 5 is typically when I start to feel the full springtime energy). This helps me plan ahead for my social life and personal relationships—now, you can do the same.

ROMANTIC RELATIONSHIPS

Now that you've come out of hibernation, inner spring will often encourage you to experiment and discover new people and activities. You'll possibly even feel flirtier here, which makes it a fun time to plan meet-ups.

Syncing your dates for the inner spring season:

❀ **Classic date:** Get tickets to a sports game. You'll be in an exciting atmosphere but still have plenty of one-on-one time with your partner.

❀ **At-home date:** Host a game night double date or group date with some of your partnered friends. Plus, you get to let the tension build for when you can be alone after the others leave.

❀ **Date with a mindful cycle twist:** At this time, you're more receptive to surprises and spontaneity. So, put a bunch of date options in a hat and just go with the flow!

In your established relationships, try adding some spontaneity in your time together. You might seek a stimulating environment like an interactive museum, or attend a wine and dinner paring at the vineyard. Since you're more playful and energetic here, you'll like the tension and connection that builds, and you might feel more experimental sexually. It's a perfect time to try something new together!

And if you're single, you'll love a night out with a few close friends. Try a new restaurant or go to a concert! If you have a potential date, plan to meet up this week since you'll be feeling social and energized.

SEX AND INTIMACY

After your period ends, you approach and enter your biologically fertile phase. Estrogen increases and you'll start to produce cervical mucus, which can make you feel wetter (even outside of sexual stimulation). Many people start this season dry, with vaginal lubrication increasing throughout spring.

For many menstruators, this is when desire picks back up. With refreshed energy and rising hormones, you may feel excited about both giving and receiving pleasure. So make time for both!

It's a prime time to experiment with new ideas and experiences around sex and intimacy. You might take a couples' massage class, try new sex toys, or read erotica. Consider what you're drawn to and vocalize the possibility of trying it out. You'll feel bolder about speaking your desires than you did in winter.

Some people may have anxiety about intercourse in this season, since most people are fertile for at least some of inner spring. The anxiety may come from the fear of potential pregnancy or the pressure to become pregnant, depending on your current life desires.

Finding a birth control method that fits your preferences and lifestyle is key. Because of my history with my IUD, I always encourage my clients to learn a FAM *alongside* their chosen form of birth control. Had I been charting my fertility signs while using an IUD, I would've caught my ectopic pregnancy before it made me lose a tube. Charting cycles can diminish pregnancy-related anxiety, whether using solely FAM for birth control or using it in conjunction with another form.

SETTING HEALTHY BOUNDARIES

Inner spring envelops us with a potent air of excitement. Harness this fun season by setting boundaries that support it.

A few boundaries my clients have set during inner spring:

- ❀ Ensuring they get in their workout before meeting up with others
- ❀ Creating an accountability chart for a new habit and hanging it up at their workspace
- ❀ Scheduling in 20 minutes a day of exploring a new hobby or idea
- ❀ Saying no to or deferring projects or goals that don't fit in with this cycle's intentions
- ❀ Reducing distractions by reminding colleagues that they're not available to meet or talk between certain hours or on certain days

INNER SUMMER: NURTURE

Your inner sun is shining, the days are long, there's a buzz in the air... Welcome to the pleasure of inner summer!

For many menstruators, inner summer is the peak of their socialness and extroversion. You're often more ambitious and flirty, and other people find you to be magnetic, too. It's a prime time to get out of your comfort zone, so use a sense of adventure when planning your time with others. If you have a hobby that includes a particular project or goal, this is where you can really push for it (and invite others to join in the fun).

Ideally, you used your inner winter and spring to prepare for this peak. By tuning into your desires in winter and by planning ahead during spring, you might have a packed but exciting schedule on your calendar. By being mindful of your needs, you can prevent the overwhelm of saying yes to events you didn't actually want to attend and choose only those obligations that truly matter to you.

ROMANTIC RELATIONSHIPS

As you're in full bloom, you'll be open to spontaneity and going with the flow. And your radiant energy can make you irresistible to others! Why not let the sparks fly?

Syncing your dates for the inner summer season:

- **Classic date:** Hit the town for dinner, drinks, and dancing. You'll feel drawn to that dance floor!

- **At-home date:** Cook a three-course meal together. You'll love the teamwork involved, and it can be extra flirty to be in the kitchen together.

- **Date with a mindful cycle twist:** You're most daring and bold around ovulation, and your physical energy peaks. So, pick an active adventure date! Go rafting, go rock climbing, or try one of those city-wide scavenger hunts.

In a committed relationship? This is your chance to do something truly exciting that will reignite the flame in your relationship. You could be drawn to high-energy environments, like dancing, outdoor adventures, or exploring a nearby city. But also look for opportunities to work as a team together, like cooking or visiting an escape room.

Single? Feel free to use this time for hands-on group activities, whether that's sports, a beach day, or a backyard barbecue. You crave social interaction at this time and are biologically wired to find a mate, if that's important to you.

SEX AND INTIMACY

Summer surrounds ovulation, and ovulation is biologically your peak time of fertility. You'll likely feel that both physically and mentally as your body prepares to release an egg! Estrogen and testosterone are at their highest. Your cervical mucus peaks in quality and quantity (increasing wetness), your cervix is high in your pelvis, and your desire may reach its maximum.

Actually, because of evolutionary biology, when you're fertile you'll naturally find yourself attracted to other people who are *not* your current partner. No need to feel guilty—this is normal and part of being a fertile human. And it's an opportunity to bring new life into your relationship.

Since you'll likely respond well to physical touch and feel that maximum desire, use your built-in seasonal boldness to ask for what you want sexually. Vocalize your needs and what you like, since your communication skills will be at their highest now. This might also be the season when you initiate intimacy more.

Feel awkward or guilty about any of that? Maybe that's your nudge to unpack any toxic beliefs you have around sex or your body. Think about that now, when you're feeling confident and connected.

You're primed for receiving pleasure when you're fertile. You might find it's easier to orgasm here, or orgasm multiple times. But it's not just about orgasms, of course! Pleasure exists in many forms. Consider bringing all five senses into your intimacy in this phase. Plus, with your increased communication skills, verbal intimacy may make you feel closer and more bonded with a partner.

SETTING HEALTHY BOUNDARIES

It's hard to say no to others during inner summer, but preparing through the other seasons will make it far easier. Your capacity for helping others is higher now, but remember to protect your own intentions and goals first.

A few boundaries my clients have set during inner summer:

❀ Setting a maximum number of social engagements per week on the calendar, and kindly saying no to additional invites

❀ Vocalizing when they're uncomfortable with somebody's words or actions, and removing themselves from the situation

❀ Putting an "unavailable" sign on the office door at work so people don't walk in with distractions (especially since those conversations may be tempting in this social season)

❀ Putting a reminder on their phone to take a full, restful lunch away from the desk

❀ Asking for a couple weeks to make a big decision (so that you can use your autumn's discernment and winter's clarity without giving in to summer's impulsiveness)

INNER AUTUMN: REFLECT

After a packed season of inner summer, your body gives you cues to slow down and close open loops.

Many people experiencing inner autumn begin to draw inward again and seek quieter, more chill experiences. It's an optimal time to focus on doing things you *truly* enjoy—not just doing them because they're there. (Ever feel FOMO—the fear of missing out? Ditch that during inner autumn.) It's good practice to balance out any social commitments with a sufficient dose of alone time, and to prioritize healthy sleep patterns as your hormones fluctuate.

Through inner summer, you could get away with a go-go-go social life, building new connections and juggling many commitments. After doing that, you'll want to recover and focus on maintaining the connections you already have. Think about what matters *most* in your relationships and act on that, instead of extra fluff. Just because you *can* doesn't mean you *have to*.

ROMANTIC RELATIONSHIPS

Autumn often grounds you back into yourself, out of the clouds of possibilities and newness. Use it as a time for the tried-and-true activities you love, with a keen eye to adjust based on your premenstrual needs.

Syncing your dates for the inner autumn season:

❀ **Classic date:** Switch up the time of day and plan a coffee or breakfast date instead of an evening one. It'll give you a feeling of productivity, and some caffeine can give you a boost to plow through the to-do list for the rest of the day. Plus, you'll be able to go to bed early to nourish your hormones.

❀ **At-home date:** Choose an activity that you can follow the steps for. Maybe it's a craft you can both try (like those step-by-step watercolor videos), or maybe it's an online wine and chocolate pairing course.

❀ **Date with a mindful cycle twist:** When the lovey-dovey hormones of ovulation have passed, you'll be more logical, practical, and in search of understanding. It might be fun to take a personality assessment together, whether it's about how you show love or what communication style you prefer. Talk about why you love those things about each other.

In an established relationship, you might not feel as excited about big adventures or nights out. Instead, prioritize the activities you already know you enjoy together. To spend meaningful time together, you might like a project that gives you a feeling of productivity or structure, like a local art class, or even actively working on your relationship.

If you're single, it's a good time to reevaluate whom you've spent time with lately. A second or third date here can give you some clarity about your true feelings, since you don't have the high of ovulation to distract you. Your critical thinking and intuition increase as well, so you'll have a better idea about what you truly think when it comes to potential relationships. Even if you make no plans to meet up, you might use your critical thinking skills to help revamp your online dating profile.

SEX AND INTIMACY

After you ovulate, estrogen takes a dip and progesterone begins to rise. Physically, your cervical mucus decreases in amount and increases in thickness. It generally feels dryer at your vulva. Your cervix is lower again after ovulation, so certain positions may feel less comfortable to you at this time.

Mentally, you may experience a decrease in sexual desire over the days. There's nothing wrong with you; it's simply evolution doing its thing. Every body is different, so take what yours says seriously.

Many menstruators crave slower sex in this season. Try turning down the speed of all intimacy, with an emphasis on foreplay. You may have easily gotten into the mood during summer but find that autumn intimacy requires a lot more time to warm up to it. Extended foreplay is an excellent practice in inner autumn to reach peak desire and pleasure. Of course, lube is a great tool, especially in these dryer days of autumn.

You may also initiate sex less, so give your partner a heads up about where you are in your cycle so they know it's natural. It's also a great time for *your* needs to be met before those of your partner. You can explain this kindly to them, so they know what will make you feel best that day, which will make them feel great, too. Maybe you'd prefer oral sex or solo sex over intercourse. Let your partner know what your hormones are saying—they can't read your mind!

Not feeling sex at the moment? It's a fantastic time to explore other types of intimacy that aren't sex. Extra cuddle sessions, deep conversations, listening to music you both love, bathing together, giving massages, enjoying a romantic dinner, kissing, writing a love note, looking at old photos, holding hands on a walk... Intimacy isn't just intercourse. The beauty of a cyclical lifestyle is allowing room for *all* kinds of pleasure.

SOME BOUNDARIES MY CLIENTS HAVE SET

❀ Setting a soft alarm half an hour before bedtime to ensure they get enough sleep

❀ Asking for a certain amount of privacy and space at home each day

❀ Delegating tasks to others when they're not their duty

❀ Kindly saying no or not this time, without giving a reason

❀ Stating that they can help someone only after they've finished the day's obligations

STRUGGLE WITH SETTING BOUNDARIES?

Let's make this clear: Boundaries are not about disconnection, punishment, or shame. They're about giving other people guidelines for how to best support you and your life.

Boundaries tell others what is important to you and what you want to protect. They give others information and feedback about maximizing your interactions together and creating a sustainable relationship.

When you don't clearly express your boundaries to others, you put both yourself and others at a disadvantage by not revealing how you can both respect each other.

CLIENT CASES: FAMILY LIFE

Heads up: I'm not currently a human parent (just a doting dog mom). But my clients have taught me how they use their cycle to support family life! A few examples:

❀ When planning activities for the kids, Cassy tries to schedule high-energy outings and events like museums and birthday parties for when she knows her energy is primed for it. During her premenstrual phase, she plans in advance for at-home activities like art projects or building blocks.

❀ Louisa hires a dog walker for a daily 30-minute walk during her inner autumn. Outsourcing even just one chore opens up space in her schedule for self-care.

❀ Joy does the bulk of the household cooking for her family, so she leans into syncing menu plans with her cycle. Apparently, her family doesn't even notice she's doing it, but it helps her feel better about her cycle and nutrition!

❀ Tanner transparently shared that although they don't have much flexibility in scheduling, they find freedom in adjusting their expectations. "When I know I have a big family commitment at a time I wouldn't have preferred to schedule it, I prepare myself by knowing it might be a different experience than I'd have planned. It's amazing when my cycle lines up energetically with my plans, since I can fully embrace it and experience it. But when it doesn't, I find ways to take care of myself before and after it, and I acknowledge that I might have to witness a different kind of energy than what's natural at that time. And that's okay!"

In all those cases, the simple self-awareness of where these parents are in their cycle gives them the grace—not guilt—to adjust plans or expectations. Remember, it's not about perfection! For most menstruators, just the awareness of the cycle makes a huge difference in mentality.

SUMMARY

How are you allowing time to recharge, connect, nurture, and reflect each cycle?

Manage your energy, not your time: Some weeks you might feel like a total extrovert, and others you'll feel like a hermit. Finding your own cyclical patterns for your social life allows you to schedule mindfully so you can be as excited as possible about your plans.

Play over perfection: Let's be real; the world isn't going to stop spinning to work with your particular cycle. It's unlikely you'll ever have even one "perfect" cycle when all your social plans, relationships, and self-care tools line up exactly with your inner seasons. So try new tools, roll with the punches, and rest assured knowing that awareness of your cycle gives you most of the benefits!

Your experience above all: Life happens. Not every cycle will have the same flow. Your season of life may change, you might see yourself see yourself totally differently from the way you did a year ago, and some relationships come while others go. Cycle syncing isn't a prescription; it's about taking note of your lived experience and applying lessons to the future.

None of us is the same person every single day. As your moods, energy, and preferences change over the course of a cycle, you can show up in your relationships and set boundaries based on what you need at that moment.

● ● ●

ENERGY + BOUNDARIES LOG

Over the next full cycle, commit to mapping out your energy and experiences within each season. Jot down a daily note or two based on the prompts for each season's chart. After the cycle completes, review your notes. What patterns did you find? What changes will you implement both with others and with yourself?

INNER SEASON LOG
(MAKE YOURSELF A COPY FOR EACH SEASON)

What tasks, people, and ideas are giving you energy right now?	
How can you add more of that into this season moving forward?	
What tasks, people, and ideas are draining your energy right now?	
What boundary could you set next cycle to lessen that?	
What social plans (if any) are appealing right now?	

INNER SEASON LOG
(MAKE YOURSELF A COPY FOR EACH SEASON)

What feels really good around love and intimacy this season?	
How can you let your partner know you want more of that in this season?	
What self-care practice feels really good this season?	
How can you incorporate a taste of that every day the next time you're in this season?	

•   •   •

THE CYCLE SYNCING HANDBOOK

CHAPTER 10

PUTTING IT ALL TOGETHER

• • •

Phew, props to you for being committed enough to your cycle to dig in this far! When you start to implement concepts and tools from all the chapters before this one, you'll likely run into a few obstacles, plus even more opportunities to individualize the way you live cyclically. Let's dig into how to approach both those challenges and chances.

WHEN YOU DON'T HAVE A TEXTBOOK CYCLE

If you have irregular cycles or perhaps don't cycle at all, you might be overwhelmed, confused, or frustrated with me right now. I get it—most of what we've covered could sound like it's for people with perfect periods. But I promise, even without a healthy or existing menstrual cycle, you can still practice cyclical living effectively and joyfully!

There are tons of factors that get in the way of normal cycles: stress, travel, pregnancy, postpartum, medications, athletic activity, malnutrition, disease, preexisting medical conditions, starting or getting off of hormonal birth control, etc. If your menstrual cycle isn't fitting neatly into four seasons, this section is for you.

WHEN YOU DON'T GET PERIODS AT ALL

If you don't currently have a menstrual cycle, you can still tune into inner seasons as a method of living cyclically. Following the moon's phases is an easy and visible tool to reference.

The moon cycle is 29.5 days, almost exactly the length of the average menstrual cycle. Call the New Moon Cycle Day 1, as if it were the start of a period; that's your inner winter. The waxing moon represents inner spring. The full moon is peak inner summer. The waning moon is inner autumn. And repeat!

Of course, you could just opt to follow a cycle over a calendar month. Instead of setting an intention on your period, you can set one on the first of every month, and proceed through your seasons from there.

Although without a true menstrual cycle, you won't experience the ups and downs of estrogen and progesterone. But remember: humans are designed to live cyclically, and even without a menstrual cycle, doing so can prevent burnout, add variety, and allow harmony across your commitments.

WHEN YOUR CYCLES ARE VERY LONG OR SHORT

Menstruators with polycystic ovarian syndrome (PCOS, a hormonal condition that leads to irregular menstrual cycles and delayed ovulation) often have a very long follicular phase (time leading up to ovulation). This can manifest as the feeling of having a lengthened but diluted inner spring. That can feel frustrating, like you feel the initial pull of spring's powers but can't quite build upon them (or they might feel exhausting after too long).

On the other hand, if you ovulate regularly but have short luteal phases (the time after ovulation), your summer might feel shortened, or you could experience short, intense autumns with bad symptoms (after all, a short luteal phase is linked to low progesterone levels).

If your ovulation is entirely unpredictable, whether due to PCOS, being postpartum, or going through perimenopause, you might feel a mix of over- and undersaturated seasons that seem to come and go without a set pattern.

Give yourself some grace in any of these situations. You might get annoyed at your cycle, and that's okay. If your menstrual cycle is frustrating you, you can opt for other methods of living cyclically, whether you choose to follow the moon phases, set daily or monthly cycles of your own, or pick and choose cyclical habits from previous chapters without them lining up with your biological phases. You can set your own inner seasons based on what will serve you most.

WHEN YOU'RE PREGNANT

When I trained as a birth and fertility doula, I was blown away by the parallels of the inner seasons to pregnancy and childbirth. If you're pregnant, you may indeed notice inner seasons that align with the childbearing process—isn't that the coolest?!

The first trimester may feel like an extended inner winter, a time to adjust to something new and fresh. You might have low energy and icky symptoms (nausea or anxiety, for example). You're changing your identity and getting in touch with your body in a new, primal way.

The second trimester brings a spring pick-me-up for many pregnant folks. Energy and appetite come back, and there's a sense of hope and possibility. This is when many people start planning a nursery, jotting down a birth plan and sharing the news with others.

Somewhere in the late second or early third trimester, people feel like they enter a summer season, a babymoon energy. Energy and mood feel stable, and you can likely still move around comfortably. Of course, the visibility piece of summer comes out with the baby bump, drawing attention. It's a time for spending time with loved ones and getting big pre-baby to-dos out of the way.

Most of the third trimester relates to an inner autumn. You might start to slow down and ask for help a lot more, especially when you feel discomfort. People find themselves nesting, batch cooking, and getting the final touches in the home ready for the baby's arrival. It's the time to set a postpartum plan and create boundaries for when the baby comes home.

Labor brings winter again—possibly the most wintery winter there is! It's the ultimate lesson in release and letting go. Laborland makes you feel distant from the world. You might feel super mammalian, looking for a dark, quiet, private space to labor. You dive into the very depths of yourself before a new being emerges.

And your winter may extend through early postpartum. They call the first three months postpartum "the fourth trimester," when rest and healing are key. Sometime after then, you'll notice an inner spring arise again, and the cycle continues.

WHEN YOU'RE GETTING OFF HORMONAL BIRTH CONTROL

Hormonal birth control interrupts the communication between your brain and ovaries. Since HBC suppresses your natural hormones, your body will need some time to start producing its own hormones and ovulating on its own again, once you stop taking HBC. For some menstruators, this happens in a month or two, for many, it takes a few months, and for an unlucky few, it could take a year or longer.

If you're stuck in a cycleless time, try living cyclically with the moon as described earlier. You can still reap the benefits of a cycle, even if your hormones aren't yet aligned. Some menstruators report that doing this encourages their natural cycles to return. It's anecdotal, of course, but doesn't hurt to try!

MAKE CYCLICAL LIVING YOUR OWN

OTHER METAPHORS FOR CYCLICAL LIVING

The four seasons are, of course, just a metaphor. You can choose another metaphor that resonates better with you, if you'd prefer. Consider hiking. You can't always be at the summit, just like you can't always stay in inner summer. You can't go downhill without going uphill, and vice versa, just like you can't have your inner autumn without your inner spring.

Or, think of the ocean tides. You might align low tide with your period, and high tide with ovulation. The rising tide may represent the same as inner spring, while the ebb current could be analogous to inner autumn.

Finally, think of one single plant in a garden. First it's a seed, then it's a sprout, then it's a bloom, and then it decays. Nature is full of cycles. Find a framework that makes sense to you and *your* cycle.

CYCLICAL DAYS

Want to live cyclically but on a daily structure? It can still be mindful and optimized to your energy patterns. Some folks find that they work through all four seasons within a full day: for example, winter is from the wind-down time before bed all the way through to the wakeup routine, spring lasts through the morning, summer is in the afternoon, and autumn takes place in the evening. You can design your day to honor your changing energy levels.

Maybe you find that morning is your best focus time for work. You can do your list-making and prioritizing while you have coffee, then dig into the most demanding work on your plate. That's your spring, and you can set spring boundaries, like using a website blocker to nix shiny distractions.

Set work categories and boundaries for the rest of your day's seasons, too. You could feel most social between noon and 4 p.m. Great—that's when you can schedule meetings, attend events, go on client calls, and run errands. After 4 p.m. might be your wind-down autumn time, when you call a friend, catch up on video recordings, and schedule creative time of some sort. Your winter

THE CYCLE SYNCING HANDBOOK

before-bed routine might involve turning off all your screens and allowing time to read.

Design your day around your daily energy levels and you might find your zest for work and life is far more sustainable than it would be if you were going in without a framework.

SEASONS OF LIFE

We've all heard someone mention the "season of life" they're in. Which season of life could you be in right now?

When I quit my job, left a relationship, and moved, I entered a long season of winter. For about one year, if I looked at my life from a bird's eye view, I felt very much in winter mode. I took a big break from working, or even planning my future at all. I kept many notes of what inspired me and new ideas I had, but I didn't put anything big into place. For me, it was all about receiving, not pushing. I embraced letting go in order to make room for the new.

At the time of writing this book, I've completed a shift into a spring season of life! I've had opportunities arise seemingly out of nowhere (though I'm now wise enough to know that they only appeared because I welcomed winter with open arms). I've been speaking to incredible audiences, hosting successful events, and finally getting clear on my next steps for my career and personal life. Even this book opportunity came to me just as I started this life season!

I anticipate that in a year or two, my life on a grand scale will be experiencing a period of inner summer. Of course, I can't predict exactly when or how or how long it'll be, but I know it will likely bring visibility, connection, and countless chances to share my gifts with the world. But I'm not in a rush. I'm enjoying this life season of spring too much.

Look back on your life so far: Can you identify large-scale seasons? Where are you right now, and how can you not only accept it, but sink into its powers?

TRANSITION DAYS

In the previous chapters, you read about signs you're transitioning into the next season. As you get more experience with noting your inner seasons, you'll begin to notice marked "transition days" that have their own particular vibe. It's like there's one foot in summer and one foot in autumn, and something about that makes you feel unbalanced, or "off."

Transition days might make you feel emotional in some way. You might get anxiety, since you've felt a hint of what's ahead. You might be resistant to the change, if you don't feel like you took advantage of the season's powers. It could feel like turbulence on a plane; you know where you're headed, but you don't feel settled in a space. You might adore certain seasonal transitions and dread others.

When you don't pay attention to your cycle, these days can catch you off guard and may even knock you off your feet. You know those weird days when you can't put a finger on why, but you feel uneasy, ungrounded, or not quite like yourself? It's much easier to anticipate and adjust when you're expecting a transition day. Note your seasonal transitions so you can plan ahead and meet yourself with self-compassion.

YOUR DEFAULT SEASON

Most of us have a season in which we feel most at home. Which season comes most easily to you? When do you feel like your most natural self? Remember, you can access that part of you at any time. It's what makes you, you!

Take note of those natural strengths, and consider what season *doesn't* come as naturally to you. Can you find a way to use your default powers to make your other seasons all a little brighter?

SHARING CYCLICAL LIVING WITH OTHERS

EXPLAINING YOUR CYCLE

The people in your life might not be used to talking about periods, and to them, cycle syncing might sound like a radical idea. When you need to explain how your cyclical life affects you, it's helpful to compare it to a concept they understand. A few ideas:

❋ **Compare it to the weather:** "To me, having my period feels like a dreary, rainy day when I just want to cozy up inside and keep to myself. When I'm ovulating, it feels like a warm, sunny day when getting out into the world is incredible. I'll need extra words of support from you on those rainy days."

❋ **Refer to the cycle of a day:** "You know how you feel super productive mid-morning and can take on all the tasks easily, but by mid-afternoon you crave a nap, and after you sleep at night, you're ready to tackle the world again? That's like how I experience a menstrual cycle."

❀ **Tell them how living cyclically benefits you:** "I've found that in the long term, I'm most productive and enthusiastic and less burned out when I approach projects from a several-weeks-long cycle rather than a day-to-day routine." Or, "I do my best proposal writing when I work from home. I'd like to suggest two days per month that I can work remotely. Is that reasonable?"

❀ **Or how it benefits others:** "I've spent some months noting my energy changes, and I know I'll be best at communicating and networking on that day. So let's plan the big presentation for then! I also know that if I ease back on drafting the slide deck this week, I'll have a superpower for making it next week."

❀ **Give them an alternative:** "I really appreciate the invite. I know I'm going to feel pretty low energy that day but really want to catch up; can we meet that Monday instead?"

❀ **Use technology:** There are apps that will sync with your partner's phone so they know where you are in your cycle and what you want and need.

❀ **Make a visual:** If your partner understands the basics, you can come up with a system to help them know what season you're in without asking. It could be a magnet on the fridge, a color-coded calendar, or a certain color of underwear!

❀ **Show them the diagram of your hormones over the course of a cycle.** 'Nuff said.

❀ **Start with the seasons!** Better yet—hand them this book.

TEAMWORK ACROSS THE SEASONS

As more menstruators start cycle syncing, the power in numbers increases. Think about a group project at work. How fantastic is it when everyone is at a different point in their cycles? You get all the powers of each season when you work together.

You can also forge alliances with cycle syncing friends. You might develop code words where the others just get it. Imagine saying, "I'll be in winter next week," and your friends already know not to make big plans or to call on you for extra help those days. Maybe you have an agreement where you walk your friend's dog when she's in her late autumn, and vice versa.

How can you take advantage of others' seasons being different from yours, and how can you share your powers with your allies when they need them?

BEFORE YOU GO OFF AND DO AMAZING THINGS

You've started down a journey, friend. Since picking up this book, you've discovered:

❀ Why cyclical living could help you live a life with more ease and joy

❀ How the four seasons parallel the four menstrual cycle phases

❀ Strategies for cycling syncing your creativity, work, movement, nutrition, relationships, and self-care

❀ How to apply cyclical wisdom even if you're not experiencing true menstrual cycles

What didn't I tell you yet? The secret fifth step of the cycle.

You know what takes place between the end of one cycle and the start of a next? *Evolution.*

Each time you experience, reflect on, and learn from a cycle, you gain a bit of inner wisdom that you'll call on in your future, whether consciously or not. It's like an upward spiral, with each completed cycle giving you an edge on living the life you want.

You'll have roughly 400 cycles in a lifetime. That's 400 chances to evolve toward your truest, most awesome self. Have fun with it. Your cycle is your superpower.

ACKNOWLEDGMENTS

• • •

When my publisher first reached out to me about potentially writing a book, I thought it might be a scam. I'd always known I'd write a book someday, yet doubts immediately crept in. "Why me? Why now? Will anyone even read this?"

Thankfully, my life bursts with infinite support from people who believe in me. I'm so grateful for those who helped bring my first book to life.

To the incredible team of life coaches I've managed to trick into befriending me over the years, Melanie McCloskey, Sarah Rosenberg Brown, and Justine Mulliez: Thank you for elevating my strengths, giving me the language to state my needs, and lifting up powerful women everywhere.

To Kelly Rusch, who introduced me to the Fertility Awareness Method: If you'd told me in high school that I'd someday write and speak about periods, I would've laughed you off the track. Endless thanks for helping me feel closer to my body than I'd ever thought possible.

To my soul sisters Katie Crafts and Jeni Stembridge: Our "Alpine Boss Babes" group was what originally gave me the confidence to launch Hormone Hacker. I'm forever grateful for the hours of inspired voice memos, magical community connections, and big escape-room energy you bring whenever we brainstorm together.

To Kudo: You taught me more than you'll ever know. Maybe dogs can't read, but whenever I look into your sweet brown eyes, I know you can feel my love for you radiating from me. Thank you for keeping my feet warm.

And to Claire Sielaff and Renee Rutledge at Ulysses Press: Thank you for answering my incessant questions, being cool enough to publish a book about periods, and embracing the freedom in my own creative process.

One book down, many to go.

ABOUT THE AUTHOR

• • •

Angie Marie is a fertility awareness educator with an adventurous edge. After a life-threatening experience with birth control convinced her to explore her reproductive options, she dove headfirst into learning all she could about pregnancy, birth and periods. After training to be a doula and then a fertility educator, Angie combined her fascination with science and her relentless creative itch to come up with resources that help menstruators make their period their superpower. An avid mountain climber and ultrarunner, Angie finds her home in the Columbia River Gorge in Washington. No matter where she's exploring, she feels her best when she's tuning into her body's wisdom. Find more menstrual cycle resources at TheHormoneHacker.com and more of Angie's work at ItsAngieMarie.com.